SMOKING

Other Books in the Current Controversies Series:

SMOKING

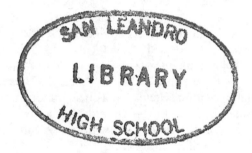

David Bender, *Publisher*
Bruno Leone, *Executive Editor*

Scott Barbour, *Managing Editor*
Brenda Stalcup, *Senior Editor*

Carol Wekesser, *Book Editor*

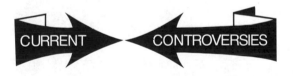

CURRENT CONTROVERSIES

Cover Photo: © Uniphoto

Library of Congress Cataloging-in-Publication Data

Smoking / Carol Wekesser, book editor.
      p. cm. — (Current controversies)
    Includes bibliographical references (p.   ) and index.
    ISBN 1-56510-534-6 (lib. bdg. : alk. paper). — ISBN 1-56510-533-8
(pbk. : alk. paper)
    1. Smoking—United States. 2. Tobacco—Health aspects. 3. Tobacco habit—United States. 4. Tobacco industry—Corrupt practices—United States. 5. Smoking—United States—Prevention. 6. Teenagers—Tobacco use—United States—Prevention. 7. Smoking—Law and legislation—United States. I. Series.
    HV5760.S663 1997
    362.29'6'0973—dc20   96-36098
                                                              CIP

Contents

in the spouses of smokers. Secondhand smoke also causes increased
respiratory problems such as asthma in the children of smokers.

Interviews and medical tests conducted over a three-year period
demonstrate that exposure to environmental tobacco smoke
(secondhand smoke) is widespread in the United States. Exposure to
such smoke is associated with numerous health problems, including
cancer, asthma, and heart disease.

Chapter 2: Is the Tobacco Industry to Blame for Leading People to Smoke?

Yes: The Tobacco Industry Is to Blame for Leading People to Smoke

Tobacco companies target their deceptive cigarette ads very
specifically to lead a variety of people to smoke. These ads imply that
cigarettes make men tougher and women thinner. Cigarette ads also
appeal to children and young teens by suggesting that smoking is a
sign of maturity. Such ads should be banned or strictly regulated.

In order to attract new customers, tobacco companies produce
advertising that targets children. Studies reveal that such ads are
effective at luring young people to smoke. Increased regulations are
needed to restrict advertising aimed at children.

New evidence reveals that the tobacco industry has worked for years
to develop tobacco with high levels of nicotine and to otherwise
control the level of nicotine delivered by cigarettes. Therefore, it can
be concluded that the tobacco industry is in the business of selling
nicotine—an addictive drug.

Many young people around the world admire the American lifestyle.
In their ads, U.S. tobacco companies play on this admiration to
persuade people in other countries to smoke their brand of cigarettes.

No: The Tobacco Industry Is Not to Blame for Leading People to Smoke

Charges that the tobacco industry has manipulated the amount of nicotine in cigarettes are untrue. Moreover, smoking is not addictive; people smoke because they choose to, not because they are nicotine addicts.

Chapter 3: How Can Smoking Be Reduced?

Chapter 4: Are Increased Measures Needed to Combat Teen Smoking?

Yes: Increased Measures Are Needed

Chapter 5: Should Government Regulation of Smoking Be Increased?

Yes: Government Regulation of Smoking Should Be Increased

Foreword

By definition, controversies are "discussions of questions in which opposing opinions clash" (Webster's Twentieth Century Dictionary Unabridged). Few would deny that controversies are a pervasive part of the human condition and exist on virtually every level of human enterprise. Controversies transpire between individuals and among groups, within nations and between nations. Controversies supply the grist necessary for progress by providing challenges and challengers to the status quo. They also create atmospheres where strife and warfare can flourish. A world without controversies would be a peaceful world; but it also would be, by and large, static and prosaic.

The Series' Purpose

The purpose of the Current Controversies series is to explore many of the social, political, and economic controversies dominating the national and international scenes today. Titles selected for inclusion in the series are highly focused and specific. For example, from the larger category of criminal justice, Current Controversies deals with specific topics such as police brutality, gun control, white collar crime, and others. The debates in Current Controversies also are presented in a useful, timeless fashion. Articles and book excerpts included in each title are selected if they contribute valuable, long-range ideas to the overall debate. And wherever possible, current information is enhanced with historical documents and other relevant materials. Thus, while individual titles are current in focus, every effort is made to ensure that they will not become quickly outdated. Books in the Current Controversies series will remain important resources for librarians, teachers, and students for many years.

In addition to keeping the titles focused and specific, great care is taken in the editorial format of each book in the series. Book introductions and chapter prefaces are offered to provide background material for readers. Chapters are organized around several key questions that are answered with diverse opinions representing all points on the political spectrum. Materials in each chapter include opinions in which authors clearly disagree as well as alternative opinions in which authors may agree on a broader issue but disagree on the possible solutions. In this way, the content of each volume in Current Controversies mirrors the mosaic of opinions encountered in society. Readers will quickly realize that there are many viable answers to these complex issues. By

11

questioning each author's conclusions, students and casual readers can begin to develop the critical thinking skills so important to evaluating opinionated material.

Current Controversies is also ideal for controlled research. Each anthology in the series is composed of primary sources taken from a wide gamut of informational categories including periodicals, newspapers, books, United States and foreign government documents, and the publications of private and public organizations. Readers will find factual support for reports, debates, and research papers covering all areas of important issues. In addition, an annotated table of contents, an index, a book and periodical bibliography, and a list of organizations to contact are included in each book to expedite further research.

Perhaps more than ever before in history, people are confronted with diverse and contradictory information. During the Persian Gulf War, for example, the public was not only treated to minute-to-minute coverage of the war, it was also inundated with critiques of the coverage and countless analyses of the factors motivating U.S. involvement. Being able to sort through the plethora of opinions accompanying today's major issues, and to draw one's own conclusions, can be a complicated and frustrating struggle. It is the editors' hope that Current Controversies will help readers with this struggle.

"Whether one views smoking as an individual choice or a physical addiction, it is a risky behavior that is difficult to quit."

Introduction

Smoking is a dangerous habit. One-fifth of all deaths in America—400,000 each year—result from smoking-related illnesses. Smoking causes 85 percent of all lung cancer deaths and contributes to one in five of all newly diagnosed cases of cancer. According to the U.S. Centers for Disease Control and Prevention, more people die from cigarette smoking and its related illnesses than die from AIDS, alcohol, traffic accidents, illicit drugs, murder, and suicide combined.

Considering these frightening statistics, it is difficult for many nonsmokers to understand why anyone would smoke. From the outsider's perspective, smoking seems unpleasant, dirty, and pointless. As the eighteenth-century writer and critic Samuel Johnson said, "Smoking . . . is a shocking thing, blowing smoke out of our mouths into other people's mouths, eyes, and noses, and having the same thing done to us."

But smoking offers some benefits: It provides a short-term energy boost, increases mental acuity, and speeds up the metabolism. Some smokers are calmed by the behaviors related to smoking—keeping their hands busy, having something in their mouths, and socializing with others who smoke.

Of those who begin smoking before the age of twenty—about 80 percent of all smokers—most cite peer pressure, rebelliousness, and curiosity as the primary reasons for taking their first puff. But once the habit is formed, many smokers say they continue smoking because they are addicted; they want to quit, but cannot. David A. Kessler, commissioner of food and drugs for the Food and Drug Administration of the Department of Health and Human Services, describes the predicament smokers face: "It is fair to argue that the decision to start smoking may be a matter of choice. But once they have started smoking regularly, most smokers are in effect deprived of the choice to stop smoking. . . . Seventeen million Americans try to quit smoking each year. But more than fifteen million individuals are unable to exercise that choice because they cannot break their addiction to cigarettes."

In 1994, the FDA concluded that cigarettes are addictive. In July 1995, the organization announced that it would seek to classify nicotine—a primary chemical in tobacco—as an addictive substance and to put the regulation of tobacco under FDA jurisdiction. (Because tobacco in the past has been considered neither food nor drug, it has not come under FDA regulation.) In August 1996, President Bill Clinton gave the FDA official approval to regulate tobacco. Such regulation could lead to stringent controls on the advertising, sale, purchase, and use of tobacco. Consequently, the tobacco industry is resisting FDA regulation through every means possible.

In their fight, representatives of the tobacco industry have strongly refuted Kessler's assertion that smoking is addictive. The industry and others who oppose FDA regulation argue that calling smoking an "addiction" is an exaggeration used by antismoking zealots to gain support for increased government control of tobacco. Mark Lender, director of advanced study and research at Kean College of New Jersey, expresses this view: "Unquestionably, many smokers find it hard to quit, but millions have quit. Exaggerated claims of addiction suggest a movement [by antismoking advocates] seeking victory at all costs." Lender and others fear that overemphasizing smoking's addictive nature will cause a push for additional government restrictions, which they say will infringe on people's freedoms. These critics of increased government control argue that regardless of tobacco's potential harms, individuals should remain free to choose whether or not to smoke.

Whether one views smoking as an individual choice or a physical addiction, it is a risky behavior that is difficult to quit. The risks and addictive potential of smoking are among the issues debated in *Smoking: Current Controversies*, which contains the following chapters: Are the Health Risks of Smoking Exaggerated? Is the Tobacco Industry to Blame for Leading People to Smoke? How Can Smoking Be Reduced? Are Increased Measures Needed to Combat Teen Smoking? Should Government Regulation of Smoking Be Increased? Throughout these chapters, authors discuss the social, economic, and physiological effects of smoking as well as the appropriate role of government in response to the continued production and consumption of cigarettes.

Chapter 1

Are the Health Risks of Smoking Exaggerated?

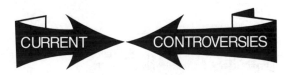

CURRENT CONTROVERSIES

The Health Risks of
Secondhand Smoke:
An Overview

by Sheryl Stölberg

About the author: *Sheryl Stölberg is the medical writer for the* Los Angeles Times *daily newspaper.*

He wanted his wife to quit smoking.

It was a simple wish, yet its consequences were profound. This was in the 1970s, in Greece, where smoking was as cherished a pastime as baseball in America. Dimitrios Trichopoulos didn't care about bucking the tide. He simply detested his wife's addiction.

A young cancer epidemiologist at the University of Athens, Trichopoulos tried the usual guilt trip. He told her she was hurting herself. On this, he said, the medical literature was clear. When that didn't work, he told her she was hurting him—an argument he could not support with statistics. She didn't believe it.

Ever the scientist, he set out to prove it.

That family argument wound up earning Trichopoulos a place in tobacco history. He was the first researcher to connect secondhand cigarette smoke with an increased risk of lung cancer.

He accomplished this in a somewhat unorthodox fashion, pirating $50,000 from one of his grants to conduct a survey of 189 nonsmoking women. (Greek officials, Trichopoulos says, would never have given him money to study the detrimental effects of a cash crop as lucrative as tobacco). He found that smokers' wives were twice as likely to develop lung cancer as women married to nonsmokers.

It worked. "I convinced her," Trichopoulos says. His wife quit.

The study did much more than clean the air in the Trichopoulos home. He published it in 1981, days before the publication of a larger study conducted by

Japanese epidemiologist Takeshi Hirayama. These papers gave a huge boost to a grass-roots anti-smoking campaign that has dramatically changed the way Americans work, dine, travel and raise children.

This is the nature of the secondhand smoke revolution: a little bit of science—still emerging, not all of it conclusive—shaping a lot of public policy.

For anti-smoking activists, scientific research into the dangers of secondhand smoke has been a godsend. The high point came in 1993, when the U.S. Environmental Protection Agency declared secondhand smoke a "Group A" human carcinogen, reporting that it accounts for 3,000 lung cancer deaths each year. This placed it in the same deadly category as asbestos and radon; the agency concluded that the danger cannot be eliminated by using smoking and nonsmoking sections.

> *"For anti-smoking activists, scientific research into the dangers of secondhand smoke has been a godsend."*

Thanks in large part to that report, secondhand smoke is now one of the nation's most pressing and divisive public health issues. Coupled with allegations that tobacco companies have misrepresented the nicotine content in cigarettes—and tobacco executives' denials—the issue is bringing public outrage to new heights.

But the tobacco industry is fighting back—hard. A coalition of farmers and manufacturers filed a lawsuit alleging that the EPA "manipulated and cherry-picked scientific data" and asked that a U.S. District Court judge in North Carolina nullify the report. In California, tobacco giant Philip Morris placed a controversial initiative on the November 1994 ballot that, if it had passed, would have invalidated local ordinances designed to curb secondhand smoke and replaced them with a looser standard.

Cigarette maker R.J. Reynolds launched an aggressive public information campaign designed to stave off smoking bans by countering the widespread perception that secondhand smoke is dangerous. The company's tactic: Fight science with science.

In full-page newspaper ads, R.J. Reynolds says its research shows that non-smokers are exposed to "very little" secondhand smoke, even when they live or work with smokers. In one month, the company said, a nonsmoker living with a smoker would breathe the equivalent of smoking 1½ cigarettes.

"Policies should be based on science," Chris Coggins, the R.J. Reynolds toxicologist, said in an interview. "I think that the [EPA] science is very, very weak."

But the industry has a long way to go toward rolling back public policy on secondhand smoke.

More than 600 state and local ordinances restrict smoking in public places, including Los Angeles' hotly debated restaurant ban. Across the United States, in cities large and small, a familiar sight has emerged: smokers congregating outside.

The federal Occupational Health and Safety Administration is contemplating a ban in all workplaces.

In May 1994, a congressional subcommittee approved a bill, introduced by Rep. Henry A. Waxman (D-Los Angeles), that would ban smoking in most buildings, except restaurants and private clubs. [The bill later died in committee.]

There is no smoking on domestic flights. There is no smoking in the White House; First Lady Hillary Rodham Clinton will not tolerate it. There is no smoking with your Big Mac; McDonald's banned tobacco in its corporate-owned restaurants. Taco Bell and Jack in the Box followed suit.

In 1993, the U.S. Supreme Court ruled in favor of a Nevada prisoner who called his cellmate's smoke cruel and unusual punishment. Custody battles have been settled by giving preference to parents who do not smoke.

The turnabout from a smoking to a smoke-free society seems to have occurred overnight. It could not have happened, anti-smoking advocates say, without science.

"Secondhand smoke is now one of the nation's most pressing and divisive public health issues."

"Twenty years ago, I tried to have one room in a cruise ship declared smoke-free and I was told I was crazy," said John Banzhaf, a law professor at George Washington University who runs Action on Smoking and Health, or ASH. "Who at that time would have figured that 30% of all our businesses would be smoke-free today? . . . Things are moving amazingly quickly, and it is the scientific, medical underpinning that has changed the complexion of the issue."

Stats Are Both Convincing and Questionable

Today, several hundred scientific studies link secondhand smoke to a variety of diseases: lung and other cancers, heart disease, respiratory infections including bronchitis and pneumonia, asthma and sudden infant death syndrome (SIDS), which claims the lives of babies as they sleep. This research is responsible for an oft-quoted statistic: About 53,000 Americans die each year from secondhand smoke.

"The evidence is so clear," says Mark Pertschuk, co-director of Americans for Non-Smokers Rights. "Everybody and his brother is lining up to ban smoking."

Yet the evidence, while compelling, is not as complete as Pertschuk suggests.

Of each year's secondhand-smoke deaths, 3,000 are attributed to lung cancer, 12,000 to other cancers and 37,000 to heart disease, according to the Coalition on Smoking OR Health, a nonprofit group formed by the American Lung Assn., the American Heart Assn. and the American Cancer Society. The coalition also estimates that secondhand smoke accounts for 700 SIDS deaths a year.

Most scientists working outside the tobacco industry say the link between lung cancer and secondhand smoke is firmly established. But the evidence on heart disease—which accounts for nearly 70% of estimated deaths—is much newer, and not all scientists accept it. Only 14 studies have documented this link, and the federal government has not yet taken a position.

Nonetheless, public tolerance for secondhand smoke is waning.

A 1994 Gallup Poll showed 38% of Americans support a ban on smoking in restaurants—up 10% from 1991. Support for workplace smoking bans is at 32%, up eight points from 1991. The poll also found 36% of Americans believe secondhand smoke is very harmful to adults, and 42% believe it is somewhat harmful.

> *"The turnabout from a smoking to a smoke-free society seems to have occurred overnight."*

"The tide has turned," says Michael Eriksen, director of the Office on Smoking and Health at the U.S. Centers for Disease Control and Prevention. "I think an invisible line was crossed in terms of how the public feels about smoking."

Vehement Opposition

The tobacco industry is trying its best to persuade people to cross back over that line.

The vast majority of the research on secondhand smoke is epidemiological, meaning it traces patterns of disease and finds connections, rather than proving cause and effect. Based on those studies, scientists are just beginning to conduct animal research to learn the precise biological effects of secondhand smoke.

Tobacco industry officials vehemently dispute the epidemiology, including the EPA report. They say some study subjects give inaccurate information about how much smoke they have been exposed to, or whether they have ever smoked.

R.J. Reynolds officials also cite a report by the Congressional Research Service—the research branch of the Library of Congress—that characterized the EPA's data as "uncertain." Coggins, the Reynolds toxicologist, complains that the EPA failed to include recent data that found no link between lung cancer and secondhand smoke.

"The epidemiological evidence is not sufficient to say that [secondhand smoke] poses a health risk," says Gio Batta Gori, a toxicologist and consultant for the Tobacco Institute, a trade industry group.

The EPA says nonsmokers face a 19% increase in their risk of developing lung cancer when they are exposed to secondhand smoke—a figure Gori describes as "a whiff of a risk." He says that if 2.5% of the study subjects misclassified themselves, the research would be invalid.

But the EPA, which estimates that 1% of subjects misclassified themselves, sticks by its findings. EPA Administrator Carol M. Browner calls the agency's science "extensively documented" and said the R.J. Reynolds ads "will not distract the public from the real issue: that secondhand smoke poses a serious health problem."

How Much Exposure?

Most independent scientists agree that secondhand smoke causes death and disease in healthy nonsmokers. It is particularly harmful to people who have underlying illnesses—asthma, heart disease, bronchitis and other respiratory conditions—that are exacerbated by cigarette fumes. But questions remain about just how much exposure will make a healthy person sick.

While living with or working near a heavy smoker is a serious health risk, the dangers of casual exposure are less clear.

"If you were a patron and you go out to eat, say, once a week, I think the disease risk may, in fact, be negligible," says Don Shopland, coordinator for the National Cancer Institute's Smoking and Tobacco Control program. "On the other hand, if you are a waitress and have to work in that environment eight hours a day for several years, you have a very substantial disease burden."

Still, Shopland says there is more than enough evidence to warrant smoking bans. He cites statistics showing that secondhand smoke–related lung cancer alone would kill 100 times as many people each year as asbestos. "And yet," he says, "if you find asbestos in a school, they will close the school."

> *"The EPA failed to include recent data that found no link between lung cancer and secondhand smoke."*

Others—including Trichopoulos— say the risks of secondhand smoke are not commensurate with the public outcry. The real health danger, they say, is to the smoker.

A smoker is 20 times more likely than a nonsmoker to develop lung cancer— a 2,000% higher risk. But, depending on the study cited, someone who breathes secondhand smoke is 1.19 times to 1.4 times as likely as a nonsmoker to develop lung cancer—a 19% to 40% higher risk.

Children Left Unprotected

There is yet another ironic twist to the way science has shaped public policy: Most laws designed to curb exposure are directed at places where adults congregate—restaurants and offices. But research shows the biggest danger is to children, particularly those whose parents smoke at home. They need the most protection, yet get the least.

According to the CDC, secondhand smoke causes up to 300,000 cases of bronchitis and pneumonia each year in children under 18 months. It can trigger or worsen asthma attacks, and may also be responsible for up to 26,000 new cases of childhood asthma each year. The agency estimates that 9 million youngsters under 5 live in homes with smokers and are exposed to secondhand smoke almost all day.

Some studies show sudden infant death syndrome is 2¹/₂ times more likely to strike babies whose mothers smoke.

These figures have been used in education campaigns, including one by the CDC and another in California financed by Proposition 99, the anti-smoking initiative adopted in 1988. Studies show the campaigns are working; people are smoking less, and are more cautious about where they smoke.

In 1993, 27% of California smokers reported they did not smoke in their homes—up from 18.8% in 1992, according to Stanton Glantz, a UC San Francisco researcher who has done extensive work on secondhand smoke. Among smokers who lived with small children, 45% said they did not smoke at home.

And no matter what the research shows, a few simple truths remain: The vast majority of American adults—76%—are not smokers. Many

> *"Questions remain about just how much exposure will make a healthy person sick."*

are annoyed by secondhand smoke. It might not make them seriously ill, but it makes their clothes smell and their eyes water. And they are no longer afraid to demand change.

The Struggle of One Researcher

For the scientists who produced what law professor Banzhaf calls the "medical underpinning" of all this social policy, the current debate is another rung on the tall ladder of acceptance. Many, like Trichopoulos, had little funding and even less support from mainstream health groups, such as the American Cancer Society and the American Heart Assn., which call secondhand smoke a major threat.

Perhaps no researcher has struggled longer or harder than James Repace. He is a 55-year-old health physicist who, while working for the Naval Research Laboratory in Washington in the late 1970s, stumbled upon the idea that secondhand smoke could be measured as air pollution. Working nights and weekends, with a borrowed air-quality monitor, he took measurements at bars, bowling alleys and office buildings.

What he found surprised him: About 85% of indoor air pollution comes from tobacco. In Repace's view, that makes secondhand smoke the biggest pollution problem in America—bigger, he says, than outdoor air pollution.

"The typical levels of particles in the air in the presence of smoking," he says, "were worse than you would find on a busy commuter highway during rush hour."

On a lark, he sent his findings to the prestigious journal *Science*. The study was published in 1980. R.J. Reynolds researcher Coggins says Repace's work relied on outdated technology. But the *Science* article helped make Repace one of the nation's leading authorities on secondhand smoke; the media often quote him and the government often uses him as an expert witness.

His success, however, has not been a boon to his EPA career.

In 1987, Repace was investigated for conflict of interest by the EPA inspector general after a Tennessee congressman complained that such outside activities prevented him from making a fair judgment about the dangers of tobacco smoke. Although he was cleared, he has been forced to leave the EPA. His bosses there, he said, have told him he is a lightning rod for complaints from the tobacco industry.

It is a conclusion that he does not dispute.

He had little to do with the landmark report declaring secondhand smoke a human carcinogen, and is "on loan" to OSHA. "At the moment," he says, "I'm looking for other things to do."

Trichopoulos' career, meanwhile, has not suffered. Today, he chairs the epidemiology department at the Harvard School of Public Health, marking him as one of the most respected researchers in his field. It has been a long journey from Greece in 1980, when, he says, he could barely get his secondhand smoke findings published.

The study finally appeared in the *International Journal of Cancer*. Trichopoulos believes that had Hirayama's study not appeared soon after in the widely read *British Medical Journal*, neither would have been taken seriously.

> **"The biggest danger is to children."**

In his Harvard office, Trichopoulos keeps a rejection letter he got from the editors of one prestigious academic journal. The letter foreshadows the political touchiness of the secondhand smoke debate. The scientist chuckles each time he reads it.

"The implications of your findings are enormous," the editors wrote. "We believe you will be proved right. . . . You will probably tell us once again that we are chicken."

Smoking Has Health Benefits

by Peter Brimelow

About the author: *Peter Brimelow is a senior editor at* Forbes, *a biweekly business magazine.*

The hangperson's noose is unmistakably around the tobacco industry's neck. In Florida and Mississippi, state governments are attempting to force tobacco companies to pay some smoking-related health care costs. In Washington, D.C., the Environmental Protection Agency has claimed that "secondhand smoke" is a significant risk for nonsmokers and the Food & Drug Administration is making noises about regulating nicotine as a drug. And the American Medical Association agreed, reasserting that nicotine is addictive. Smokers have already been driven from many workplaces into the street for a furtive puff. But further legal harassment, to the point of what an industry spokesman calls "backdoor prohibition," seems unstoppable.

The Rewards of Smoking

Lost in this lynching frenzy: the fact that smoking might be, in some small ways, good for you.

Hold on now! Let's be clear: *The Surgeon General has* indeed *determined that smoking is dangerous to your health*. Lung cancer and cardiovascular diseases are highly correlated with cigarette consumption. Annual smoking-related deaths are commonly said to be over 400,000 (although critics say the number is inflated).

But so is driving automobiles dangerous to your health (over 40,000 deaths a year). Yet people do it, because it has rewards as well as risk. And they judge, as individuals, that the reward outweighs the risk.

This is called freedom.

Well, what are the rewards of cigarette smoking? Apart from intangible pleasure, the most obvious is behavioral. A battery of studies, such as those by

Peter Brimelow, "Thank You for Smoking. . . ?" *Forbes*, July 4, 1994. Reprinted by permission of *Forbes* magazine, © Forbes Inc., 1994.

British researcher D.M. Warburton, show that cigarettes, whatever their other effects, really do stimulate alertness, dexterity and cognitive capacity.

And alertness, dexterity, etc. can be useful. Such as when driving. Or flying—as Congress recognized when it exempted airline pilots from the ban on smoking on domestic flights.

These behavioral benefits suggest an answer to the Great Tobacco Mystery: why almost a third of adult Americans continue to do something they are told, incessantly and insistently, is bad for them. (Duke University economist W. Kip Viscusi reported in his 1992 book, *Smoking: Making the Risky Decision*, that survey data show smokers, if anything, exaggerate the health danger of their habit.)

Smokers, according to numerous studies such as those by University of Michigan researchers Ovide and Cynthia Pomerleau, are different from nonsmokers. They tend toward depression and excitability. Current understanding is that nicotine is "amphoteric"—that is, it can act to counter both conditions, depending on how it is consumed. (Quick puffs stimulate, long drags calm.)

The implication is fascinating: A large part of the population seems to be aware of its significant although not pathological personality quirks, and to have discovered a form of self-medication that regulates them.

Other Health Benefits

Of course, this explanation for the stubbornness of smokers is not as satisfying as what Washington prefers to believe: mass seduction by the wicked tobacco companies and their irresistible advertising. Nor would it justify huge rescue operations by heroic politicians and bureaucrats.

Beyond its behavioral effects, smoking seems also to offer subtler health rewards to balance against its undisputed risks:

• *Parkinson's disease.* The frequency of this degenerative disorder of the nervous system among smokers appears to be half the rate among nonsmokers—an effect recognized by the Surgeon General as long ago as 1964.

• *Alzheimer's disease.* Similarly, the frequency of this degenerative mental disorder has recently been found to be as much as 50% less among smokers than among nonsmokers—for example, by the 11 studies reviewed in the *International Journal of Epidemiology* in 1991.

> *"Smoking might be, in some small ways, good for you."*

• *Endometrial cancer.* There is extensive and long-standing evidence that this disease of the womb occurs as much as 50% less among smokers—as documented by, for example, a *New England Journal of Medicine* article back in 1985. The triggering mechanism appears to be a reduction in estrogen levels.

• *Prostate cancer.* Conversely, smoking seems to raise estrogen levels in men and may be responsible for what appears to be a 50% lower rate of prostate cancer among smokers, although this needs corroboration.

• *Osteoarthritis.* This degenerative disorder of bone and cartilage is up to five times less likely to occur among heavy smokers—as documented, for example, by the federal government's first Health and Nutrition Examination Survey.

• *Colon cancer, ulcerative colitis.* These diseases of the bowel seem to be about 30% and 50% less frequent among smokers—documented, for example, by articles in the *Journal of the American Medical Association* and in the *New England Journal of Medicine* in 1981 and 1983, respectively.

Other benefits that have been suggested for smoking: lower rates of sarcoidosis and allergic alveolitis, both lung disorders, and possibly even acne. Smokers are also lighter—ironic, because obesity is a leading cause of the cardiovascular disease that smoking is also supposed to exacerbate. So you could quit smoking and still die of a heart attack because of the weight you put on.

None of these health benefits is enough to persuade doctors to recommend occasional cigarettes, in the way that some now occasionally recommend a glass of wine.

But consider this theoretical possibility: Should 60-year-olds take up smoking because its protection against Alzheimer's is more immediate than its potential damage to the lungs, which won't show up for 30 years if at all?

A theoretical possibility—and likely to remain theoretical. Research into possible benefits of tobacco and nicotine is widely reported to be stymied by the absolutist moral fervor of the antismoking campaign.

An All-Out War

Under the Carter Administration, the federal government abandoned its research into safer cigarettes in favor of an attack on all smoking. No effort is made to encourage smokers to switch to pipes and cigars, although their users' lung cancer and heart disease rates are five to ten times lower (somewhat offset by minor increases in mouth and throat cancers). There is no current support for studies of the marginal increase in danger for each cigarette smoked, although it appears the human system can clear the effects of three to five of the (much stronger) pre-1960 cigarettes, if dispersed across a day, with relatively little risk.

Instead, the extirpation of smoking has become another "moral equivalent of war"—as President Carter called the energy crisis in the 1970s, and as price and wage controls were viewed earlier. There is no role for tradeoffs, risk-reward calculations or free choice.

Why don't tobacco companies point out the potential offsetting rewards of smoking? Besides the usual corporate cowardice and bureaucratic inertia, the answer may be another, typically American, disease—lawyers. Directing the companies' defense, they apparently veto any suggestion that smoking has benefits for fear of liability suits and of the possible regulatory implications if nicotine is seen as a drug.

Which leaves smokers defenseless against a second typically American disease: the epidemic of power-hungry puritanical bigots.

The Health Risks of Secondhand Smoke Are Exaggerated

by W. Kip Viscusi

About the author: *W. Kip Viscusi is the George G. Allen Professor of Economics at Duke University in Durham, North Carolina.*

The regulation of public smoking has become an increasingly prominent policy issue. Many public and private institutions have instituted policies to restrict public smoking. Some have banned public smoking altogether. At a governmental level, the Occupational Safety and Health Administration (OSHA) has proposed banning all public smoking in the workplace, except for smoking in lounges that meet highly restrictive requirements. Recently the U.S. Environmental Protection Agency (EPA) also issued a report in support of legislation banning all public smoking.

The debate over taxing cigarettes has intensified as well. Advocates of higher cigarette taxes cite the health care costs inflicted by smokers on the rest of society. In 1994, for example, the proposed Clinton health care plan included a tax of 99¢ per pack of cigarettes, and a health care bill from the House Education and Labor Committee would have imposed a tax of $2.00 a pack. Unlike smoking restrictions of various kinds, taxes are targeted mechanisms for addressing societal costs associated with environmental tobacco smoke (ETS) [or secondhand smoke], as opposed to reducing smoking more generally.

Costs and Benefits

Smoking restrictions are a sensible and appropriate policy tool for limiting exposure to cigarette smoke. However, that does not mean that all public smoking should be banned. The key policy issues are how broad such public smoking restrictions should be and who should have the responsibility for setting the restrictions. As with all regulatory policies, the overall benefits to society from

Excerpted from W. Kip Viscusi, "Secondhand Smoke: Facts and Fantasy," *Regulation*, no. 3, 1995. Reprinted by permission of the Cato Institute.

such efforts should exceed the costs they generate.

As the percentage of nonsmokers in society has risen, the expectations of nonsmokers with respect to anti-smoking policies have steadily risen. Consider the following Gallup Poll results. In 1978 only 43 percent of all respondents believed that smoking on commercial airplanes should be banned completely. Similarly, in 1977 only 16 percent of respondents believed that smoking in public places should be banned. By 1987 the fraction of respondents supporting a complete ban on smoking in all public places had risen to 55 percent, and in 1988 it reached 60 percent. Within the course of only a decade there was dramatic surge in the strength of public support for smoking restrictions.

> *"The case for banning smoking in the workplace on risk-based grounds is not compelling."*

The presence of ETS is a classic externality problem. Smokers derive pleasure from their smoking activity, but it gives rise to a side effect that is undesirable for those exposed to the smoke. Clearly, we can restrict smoking activity, but doing so will decrease the welfare of smokers. How should we think about regulating smoking, and what is the appropriate extent of the regulation?

The Risks of Environmental Tobacco Smoke

For many years nonsmokers viewed ETS as a smelly annoyance. Recently the stakes have been raised as opponents of smoking have begun to characterize ETS as a threat to individual health. The health dimension has changed the terms of the debate, greatly increasing the moral authority that nonsmokers are bringing to bear. It is therefore useful to inquire whether ETS is in fact a major threat to the health of nonsmokers.

Cancer researchers generally note that the body is resilient in the presence of some carcinogens. One whiff of ETS is proportionately less likely to be risky than massive and sustained exposures. Government agencies such as the EPA and OSHA have not made such distinctions. . . . It is nevertheless instructive to assess the extent of the risks that the agencies have estimated. It should be noted at the outset that the consensus among economic researchers, including the Congressional Research Service, is that the state of science with respect to ETS is too uncertain to warrant estimation of the health consequences.

There are two classes of health hazards that have been linked to ETS: lung cancer and heart disease. Most of the public discussion has focused on the lung cancer estimates, whereas the heart disease estimates are both more speculative and much larger in magnitude. Let us consider each of these in turn.

Lung Cancer

The EPA's assessment of the lung cancer risks was based on a review of 11 studies of family members exposed to ETS. Only one of the 11 studies indicated statistically significant effects . . . , and in some cases the influences were in the "wrong" direction. Such statistically significant results can occur on a random basis. Rather than dismissing the linkages as not well established, the EPA averaged the implications of the studies to obtain a risk estimate. OSHA reviewed the same set of studies and applied different weights to derive a somewhat lower risk estimate.

The scientific studies used for the EPA and OSHA risk assessments in no way adjusted for the changing character of the cigarettes between the time of exposure and the current period, when tar levels in cigarettes are much reduced. In addition, studies of household members, as in all existing ETS studies, involve individuals exposed to much greater concentrations and longer durations of cigarette smoke than in public smoking contexts. . . .

More fundamentally, the studies failed to include the usual kind of . . . controls that are the norm in economic analysis. Smokers who choose to live in polluted areas or who are married to other smokers will tend to incur nonsmoking risks correlated with ETS because of a difference in risk-taking propensities. For example, my past research with Joni Hersch of the University of Wyoming has established that cigarette smokers and those who do not wear seatbelts are much more willing to work at hazardous jobs. A higher cancer risk for family members of smokers would be consistent with that type of pattern.

In terms of an overall cancer estimate, the EPA estimates that each year 2,200 people die from ETS exposures. Overall, 1,694 deaths are caused by exposures outside of the home. In the OSHA estimates of the risk levels, the total number of ETS deaths outside the home ranges from a lower bound of 444 to an upper bound of 1,150. Focusing solely on the workplace, the OSHA ETS risk range is from 171 to 880 lung-cancer deaths per year. . . .

Heart Disease

The estimates of heart disease costs associated with ETS are considerably higher. The EPA estimates that 8,760 to 17,520 heart disease deaths per year are attributable to ETS. The estimates are based on a single study in the literature, a study that is replete with caveats made by the author, such as the following: "While the lung-cancer risk among never-smokers exposed to ETS is well established, a possible risk of heart disease due to ETS is more controversial. . . . There are many risk factors for heart disease, and it is difficult to control well for all of them. . . . A number of assumptions are involved in estimating the disease mortality due to ETS, adding an unfortunate level of uncertainty."

"There are more important and fundamental threats to workers' lives than ETS."

Perhaps the most important deficiency of the EPA and OSHA estimates is that the risk estimates for heart disease induced by ETS are implausibly large relative to the lung cancer risks for ETS, and given the direct estimates of the heart disease risk and other risks to the smokers themselves. Personal characteristics, which are likely to be correlated with risk and the social status of smokers, were omitted from the analysis.

Are the Risks Significant?

In justifying its regulatory initiative with respect to public smoking in the workplace, OSHA maintains that it is obligated by its enabling legislation and related court decisions to regulate all "significant" risks. OSHA concludes that the lung cancer risks alone, which are the better established of the ETS risks, are significant, and consequently merit regulation. Since OSHA's interpretation of its regulatory mandate differs from the usual economic prescription that agencies should take a balanced view and pursue regulations that are in society's overall best interest, recognizing both benefits and costs, it is instructive to examine this risk-based rationale more closely.

> *"The substantial publicity given to ETS issues may have led to exaggerated risk perceptions."*

In terms of the statistical significance of the effects, 10 of the 11 studies cited to justify the regulation fail to indicate a statistically significant linkage. But is the magnitude of the effects substantial, although perhaps not precisely established? In the 1980 OSHA *Benzene* case (*AFL-CIO v. American Petroleum Institute*), the Supreme Court indicated that a one in a billion risk from drinking chlorinated water would not be considered significant, but a one in a thousand risk from gasoline vapors would be significant. Are the risks from ETS significant?

To answer that question, OSHA took a lifetime risk perspective, and it is useful to apply that approach to the Supreme Court's view that a one in a billion risk from chlorinated water would not be significant. The amount of water people drink per day from different sources ranges from 2.1 to 2.9 quarts. To be conservative, I will assume that people drink nine glasses of chlorinated water per day (that may come, for example, from sodas or other products). The individual who drinks nine glasses per day each year for 70 years will drink 229,950 glasses during his lifetime. If the risk per glass is one in a billion, as hypothesized by the Court, the lifetime risk is two in ten thousand.

Now let us consider ETS. OSHA estimates that between 144 and 722 people will die from lung cancer each year because of ETS. If the 74 million nonsmoking American workers exposed to ETS are exposed over their entire 40-year employment expectancy, their lifetime risk ranges from one in ten thousand to four in ten thousand. Thus, the risk of drinking chlorinated water falls between the two bounds of the risk range estimated by OSHA for ETS. When translated into lifetime risks as opposed to risks from a particular exposure, so that both the ETS risks and the chlorinated water risks being discussed by the Court are in the same time dimension, we find that the risks are quite comparable and are of the same general magnitude.

Even if the flawed scientific evidence is taken at face value, the case for banning smoking in the workplace on risk-based grounds is not compelling. Quite simply, there are more important and fundamental threats to workers' lives than ETS. That does not mean that ETS should not be a matter of concern, but rather that one should take a balanced view and assess the overall merits of such regulation.

The Role of Market Forces

The market will in fact respond to ETS as it does in the case of other environmental amenities. After all, ETS is not the only aspect of the restaurant business that partakes of a public goods character; others include the music that is played and the general ambiance of the restaurant. If the restaurant is unpleasant, whether it be because the music is too loud or the ETS is annoying to nonsmokers, the customers will go elsewhere. Restaurants in turn will establish nonsmoking areas, since they have a financial interest in keeping their nonsmoking customers.

"An exaggerated perception of the risk will lead to excessive restrictions on smoking in the workplace."

A similar kind of phenomenon occurs in the workplace. If workers perceive their exposures to ETS as unpleasant or risky, they will demand [compensation] for those exposures. The resulting costs will in turn raise the cost to the employer of hiring smokers. Company responses may include the provision of smoking lounges or instituting local smoking restrictions in contexts where they are appropriate. One would expect such private bargains to be more balanced than regulations such as those initiated by OSHA, since the decisionmaker has an incentive to reflect on the consequences of the smoking restrictions both for smokers and nonsmokers.

Assessing Risks

For private-sector responses to work, there must be information to enable the parties to make sound decisions. To the extent that ETS has an unpleasant odor, this is a readily monitorable attribute. However, the potential risks associated with smoking are less easily assessed. Although risk perceptions may not be perfect, the nature of the systematic bias is that as a whole, people tend to overestimate the risk level. The direction of the bias is consequently the opposite of what would be needed to have a market failure that warrants government intervention.

In my past research, I have shown that the average American adult assesses the risk of lung cancer from smoking to be 0.43, far above the estimates based on the surgeon general reports that peg the risk at between 0.05 and 0.10. Similarly, people overestimate the overall smoking-mortality risk level, which they believe to be 0.54. In contrast, estimates based on the reports by the U.S. surgeon general peg that risk in the range of 0.18 to 0.36. People assess life expectancy loss from smoking as 11.5 years, which also greatly exceeds the estimated life expectancy loss based on available scientific evidence.

The ETS risks are also likely to be overestimated because of the substantial publicity they have received. The current public debate over smoking and ETS involves prominent officials from the EPA, OSHA, and the FDA [Food and Drug Administration]. Most workers are aware of the ETS debate. Indeed, OSHA cites evidence indicating that "88 percent of nonsmokers are aware of the negative health consequences of ETS." The substantial publicity given to ETS issues may have led to

> *"What is needed is a rational assessment of the risks."*

exaggerated risk perceptions. The literature on the economics and psychology of risk perception clearly documents that highly publicized risks tend to be overestimated. The potential hazards of smoking are among the most highly publicized and widely discussed risks in our society.

The implication . . . is that the market response to the risk of smoking may in fact be excessive. Rather than leading to too little market accommodation of the preferences of nonsmokers, an exaggerated perception of the risk will lead to excessive restrictions on smoking in the workplace. Thus, it may be the case that the actions that have been undertaken are already too stringent from the standpoint of their overall social desirability.

Restrictions on workplace smoking are already quite widespread. A 1991 survey of company smoking policies found that 85 percent of all firms had smoking policies. Of those policies, 34 percent were bans, and another 34 percent involved prohibition of smoking in all open work areas. Moreover, over 90 percent of nonmanufacturing establishments also had smoking policies. As one might expect, smoking policies are more common in larger establishments than in smaller enterprises. . . .

Thinking About Smoking Restrictions

The anti-smoking fervor has led to the support of a variety of initiatives that would dramatically restrict public smoking. The linchpin of those efforts has been the estimated health impact of ETS on nonsmokers. However, the existence of health effects has led many participants in the debate to lose sight of the competing interests involved.

The existing scientific evidence is highly speculative. Existing studies focus only on exposure of other household members and fail to control adequately for household characteristics correlated with a smoking spouse that may lead to risks of lung cancer and heart disease. What is needed is a rational assessment of the risks, rather than an advocacy perspective from either side. Instead of focusing on worst-case scenarios, we should be seeking out the best available scientific evidence. Available scientific studies may not be conclusive, but that fact alone should not necessarily be a rationale for inaction. On the other hand, we should not be swayed by fragmentary evidence that is inconsistent with other, better-established relationships, such as the magnitude of the risks to smokers themselves.

Regardless of which ETS risk estimates one employs, the ETS costs to society are clearly not infinite. Indeed, if we calculate the costs of ETS as well as the other insurance-related costs generated by smokers, cigarette smokers still pay their own way, given the taxes they pay for consuming the product. The financial merits of the case . . . in no way justify restrictions on public smoking.

That is not to say that some form of smoking regulation in particular contexts would not be desirable. Nonfinancial concerns are also relevant. However, when we examine the desirability of smoking regulations, we should recognize the competing effects such efforts have. Smokers lose a substantial benefit to their welfare by having their smoking activity restricted, and losses accrue to society in terms of foregone taxes. Companies suffer foregone profits. There are also direct costs of restrictions, such as the expense associated with setting aside smoking areas and the possible productivity loss from impeding smoking behavior.

In many contexts, the market is well equipped to deal with such tradeoffs by reflecting the competing costs and benefits of restricting smoking. Indeed, most enterprises in the United States have enacted smoking-related policies. Provided that such efforts are not motivated by excessive reactions to publicity associated with ETS, they will be well founded.

For the government to promulgate sound regulations, it should follow the same kind of thought process that would be adopted in the market. Indeed, a useful starting point would be for there to be an assessment of which situations the market will not deal with adequately, since otherwise there is no need for government intervention. In any event, there is a need for reason and balance in recognition of the welfare consequences of smoking restrictions, not only for nonsmokers but for smokers and society at large.

Smoking Is Harmful to Human Health

by William F. Harrison

About the author: *William F. Harrison is an obstetrician and a gynecologist in Fayetteville, Arkansas.*

Most of us in medicine now accept that tobacco is associated with major health consequences and constitutes the No. 1 health problem in this country.

Complications of Smoking

What smokers have not yet come to terms with is that if they continue smoking, the probability of developing one or more of the major complications of smoking is 100%. It absolutely will happen. They will develop chronic bronchitis, laryngitis, pharyngitis, sinusitis and some degree of emphysema. It is also highly probable that they will develop serious disease in the arteries of all vital organs, including the brain and heart, markedly increasing their risk of heart attack and stroke. If they continue, they increase the probability of developing cancer of the lips, gums, tongue, pharynx, larynx, trachea, bronchi and lungs, of the bladder, cervix, gallbladder and other organs. Smoking contributes to rapid aging of the skin and connective tissues—women and men who smoke usually have the skin age of a person 10 to 20 years older than one who doesn't smoke, given the same degree of exposure to the sun.

About 415,000 people die prematurely each year in the U.S. as a result of smoking—the equivalent of eighteen 747s' crashing every week with no survivors. Many of these victims die after long and excruciating illnesses, burdens to themselves, their families and society. The cost of this misery is incalculable, but we do know that the tobacco industry grosses about $50 billion a year from the agonies it inflicts.

How does all this damage come about?

In normal lungs, the trachea and bronchi—the large and small tubes leading to the alveoli (the tiny sacs that do the actual work of the lungs)—are lined with

William F. Harrison, "Why Stop Smoking? Let's Get Clinical," *Los Angeles Times*, July 7, 1996. Reprinted with permission.

a film of tissue that is one cell layer thick. The surface of these cells is covered with tiny, finger-like structures called cilia. These cilia beat constantly in a waving motion, which moves small particles and toxic substances out of the lung and into the back of the throat where they are swallowed. In a smoker or someone like a coal miner, who constantly breathes in large amounts of toxic substances, many of the cilia soon disappear. If exposure continues, some ciliated cells die and are replaced by squamous cells, the same

> *"About 415,000 people die prematurely each year in the U.S. as a result of smoking."*

type that form the skin. Without the cleansing function of the ciliated cells, toxic materials and particles are breathed further into the lungs, staying longer in contact with all the tissue. Each group of ciliated cells killed and replaced by squamous cells decreases by a certain fraction the lungs' ability to cleanse themselves. As this occurs, the amount of damage done by each cigarette increases to a greater and greater degree. By the time one has been a pack-a-day smoker for 10 years or so, extensive damage has already been done. By 20 years, much of the damage is irreversible and progresses more rapidly. After 10 years of smoking, each cigarette may do as much damage to the body as three or more packs did when a smoker first started.

The longer one smokes, the harder it gets to quit. Smoking is one of the most addictive of human habits, perhaps as addicting as crack cocaine or heroin. One has to quit every day, and there are no magic pills or crutches that make stopping easy. It is tough to do. Only those who keep trying ever quit. And even those who have smoked for only a short time or few cigarettes a day will probably find it difficult to stop. But the sooner a smoker makes this self-commitment, the more probable it is that he or she will quit before having done major damage to the body.

Nicotine Is Extremely Addictive

by David A. Kessler

About the author: *David A. Kessler is the commissioner of the U.S. Food and Drug Administration of the U.S. Department of Health and Human Services.*

The cigarette industry has attempted to frame the debate on smoking as the right of each American to choose. The question we must ask is whether smokers really have that choice.

Consider these facts:

- Two-thirds of adults who smoke say they wish they could quit.
- Seventeen million try to quit each year, but fewer than one out of ten succeeds. For every smoker who quits, nine try and fail.
- Three out of four adult smokers say that they are addicted. By some estimates, as many as 74 to 90 percent are addicted.
- Eight out of ten smokers say they wish they had never started smoking. . . .

The Grip of Nicotine

The nicotine delivered by tobacco products is highly addictive. This was carefully documented in the 1988 Surgeon General's report. You can find nicotine's addictive properties described in numerous scientific papers.

As with any addictive substance, some people can break their addiction to nicotine. But I doubt there is a person who hasn't either gone to great pains to quit smoking, or watched a friend or relative struggle to extricate himself or herself from a dependence on cigarettes.

Remarkably, we see the grip of nicotine even among patients for whom the dangers of smoking could not be starker. After surgery for lung cancer, almost half of smokers resume smoking. Among smokers who suffer a heart attack, 38 percent resume smoking while they are still in the hospital. Even when a smoker has his or her larynx removed, 40 percent try smoking again.

When a smoker sleeps, blood levels of nicotine decrease significantly. But the

From David A. Kessler, "Statement on Nicotine-Containing Cigarettes" to the House Committee on Energy and Commerce, Subcommittee on Health and the Environment, March 25, 1994.

smoker doesn't need to be an expert on the concept of nicotine blood levels to know full well what that means. More than one-third of smokers reach for their first cigarette within 10 minutes of awakening; nearly two-thirds smoke within the first half hour. Experts in the field tell us that smoking the first cigarette of the day within 30 minutes of waking is a meaningful measure of addiction.

Young People

I am struck especially by the statistics about our young people. A majority of adult smokers begin smoking as teenagers. Unfortunately, 70 percent of young people ages 12–18 who smoke say that they believe that they are already dependent on cigarettes. About 40 percent of high school seniors who smoke regularly have tried to quit and failed.

It is fair to argue that the decision to start smoking may be a matter of choice. But once they have started smoking regularly, most smokers are in effect deprived of the choice to stop smoking. Recall one of the statistics I recited earlier. Seventeen million Americans try to quit smoking each year. But more than 15,000,000 individuals are unable to exercise that choice because they cannot break their addiction to cigarettes. My concern is that the choice that they are making at a young age quickly becomes little or no choice at all and will be very difficult to undo for the rest of their lives.

An Addictive Substance

Nicotine is recognized as an addictive substance by such major medical organizations as the Office of the U.S. Surgeon General, the World Health Organization, the American Medical Association, the American Psychiatric Association, the American Psychological Association, the American Society of Addiction Medicine, and the Medical Research Council in the United Kingdom. All of these organizations acknowledge tobacco use as a form of drug dependence or addiction with severe adverse health consequences.

Definitions of an addictive substance may vary slightly, but they all embody some key criteria: first, compulsive use, often despite knowing the substance is harmful; second, a psychoactive effect—that is, a direct chemical effect in the brain; third, what researchers call reinforcing behavior that conditions continued use. In addition,

> *"For every smoker who quits, nine try and fail."*

withdrawal symptoms occur with many drugs and occur in many cigarette smokers who try to quit. These are hallmarks of an addictive substance and nicotine meets them all.

Animal Studies

When a smoker inhales, once absorbed in the bloodstream, nicotine is carried to the brain in only 7–9 seconds, setting off a biological chain reaction that is critical in establishing and reinforcing addiction.

Over the past few years, scientists have generated a tremendous amount of information on the similarities among different addictive substances. Some crucial information has come from the fact that, in a laboratory setting, animals will self-administer addictive substances. This self-administration may involve the animal pushing a lever or engaging in other actions to get repeated doses of the addictive substance. With very few exceptions, animals will self-administer those drugs that are considered highly addictive in humans, including morphine and cocaine, and will not self-administer those drugs that are not considered addictive.

> *"The nicotine delivered by tobacco products is highly addictive."*

Understanding that animals will self-administer addictive substances has fundamentally changed the way that scientists view addiction in humans. It has turned attention away from the concept of an "addictive personality" to a realization that addictive drugs share common chemical effects in the brain.

Despite the wide chemical diversity among different addictive substances, a property that most of them share is the ability to affect the regulation of a chemical called dopamine in parts of the brain that are important to emotion and motivation. It is now believed that it is the effect of addictive substances on dopamine that is responsible for driving animals to self-administer these substances and for causing humans to develop addictions.

Regulation of dopamine rewards the activity, and causes the animal or person to repeat the activity that produced that reward. The process by which the regulation of dopamine leads an animal or a human to repeat the behavior is known as "reinforcement." Drugs that have the ability to directly modify dopamine levels can produce powerfully ingrained addictive behavior.

Little Pleasure in Smoking

One of the ways that researchers now test the addictive properties of drugs is to determine whether animals will self-administer that substance and then to determine whether the animals will stop self-administering if the chemical action of the substance is blocked by the simultaneous administration of another drug that prevents the first substance from acting in the brain. Data gathered over the past 15 years have documented that laboratory animals will voluntarily self-administer nicotine; that nicotine does stimulate the release of dopamine; and that laboratory animals will decrease self-administration of nicotine if the action of nicotine, or the release of dopamine, in the brain is blocked.

A number of top tobacco industry officials have stated that they do not believe that tobacco is addictive. They may tell you that smokers smoke for "pleasure," not to satisfy a nicotine craving. Experts tell us that their patients report that only a small minority of the cigarettes they smoke in a day are highly pleasurable. Experts believe that the remainder are smoked primarily to sustain nicotine blood levels and to avoid withdrawal symptoms.

The industry couches nicotine's effects in euphemisms such as "satisfaction" or "impact" or "strength." Listen to what they say in one company's patent:

> It also has been generally recognized that the smoker's perception of the "strength" of the cigarette is directly related to the amount of nicotine contained in the cigarette smoke during each puff.

But these terms only sidestep the fact that the companies are marketing a powerfully addictive agent. Despite the buzzwords used by industry, what smokers are addicted to is not "rich aroma" or "pleasure" or "satisfaction." What they are addicted to is nicotine, pure and simple, because of its psychoactive effects and its drug dependence qualities.

To smokers who know that they are addicted, to those who have buried a loved one who was addicted, it is simply no longer credible to deny the highly addictive nature of nicotine.

Secondhand Smoke Threatens the Health of Americans

by Elizabeth M. Whelan

About the author: *Elizabeth M. Whelan is the president of the American Council on Science and Health, an association of scientists and doctors concerned with public health.*

In 1993, the Environmental Protection Agency released its long awaited report assessing the health risks of other people's cigarette smoke—"Environmental Tobacco Smoke (ETS)." Their conclusion: ETS causes 3,000 cases of lung cancer annually in nonsmokers; it is responsible for hundreds of thousands of cases of bronchitis and pneumonia in children; and it induces or worsens asthma in up to one million young Americans. The public health community welcomed the official findings—noting they were consistent with other scientific reviews.

The tobacco industry—which has, for over 40 years, been blowing smoke by officially dismissing the causal link between active smoking and premature disease and death—responded with denials and accusations that the EPA study was the product of a fanatical anti-smoking movement that was manipulating data to advance their ultimate agenda: universal restrictions on smoking. The industry filed suit against the EPA in federal court in Greensboro, North Carolina, requesting that the judge declare the classification of ETS as a "Class A" carcinogen "null and void."

Science or Fiction

Is there scientific evidence that passive or second-hand smoke is a health hazard? Or is the EPA conclusion yet another example of government-inspired "science fiction" engineered, in this case, by those who are waging an ideological vendetta against the tobacco industry?

Elizabeth M. Whelan, "Is Secondhand Smoke *Really* a Threat to Our Health?" Reprinted with permission from *Priorities* (Fall/Winter 1993), a publication of the American Council on Science and Health, 1995 Broadway, 2nd Floor, New York, NY 10023-5860.

Scientific credibility: The EPA has a dismal record in separating real health risks from bogus ones. It was this agency which slapped the designation "probable human carcinogen" on the apple growth regulator, Alar, in 1989 and contributed to the great Apple Panic. The Alar apple scare was later shown to be scientifically baseless. The EPA oversees the Superfund program which targets "cancer causing" dumpsites. Yet, there is no evidence that such sites pose any cancer risk at all. It was the EPA that called for the evacuation of Times Beach, Missouri, at a cost of about $20 million, touting the hypothetical risk of dioxin.

So when EPA calls ETS a "Class A carcinogen" (meaning there is human evidence that it causes cancer), skeptics from both the business and scientific communities (myself included) wondered if this was not just more environmental hype. But, just as past crimes cannot be considered as evidence in a current trial, we cannot judge the EPA because it has overstated or misrepresented risks in the past. We must judge them on the current facts.

Plausibility: Theoretically, one could advance the opinion that anything—say fax machines or Kleenex—causes cancer. But to be taken seriously, such claims need a biological hypothesis, a scientific context in which they make sense. Clearly, the hypothesis that ETS causes human cancer *does* have that biological context. Second-hand smoke has essentially the same chemical components as direct smoke—and we know beyond any reasonable doubt that direct smoke dramatically increases the risk of cancer of the lung, bladder, pancreas, cervix, esophagus and other sites. Active smoking increases cancer risk even at low exposure, five to ten cigarettes per day, a level of carcinogen exposure that may be in the same range as high dose ETS exposure. (At least one published autopsy study confirmed that nonsmokers married to smokers frequently have precancerous lesions on their lungs.) But, is there evidence that ETS is present at sufficiently high doses to cause cancer? (The argument that passive inhalation is less hazardous than primary smoking because smoke gets filtered through the nose rather than being taken directly into the lungs from the mouth has now been dismissed because researchers have found that ETS particles are so small that they escape the nasal filtering system and also directly enter the lungs.)

> *"Nonsmokers married to smokers frequently have precancerous lesions on their lungs."*

Exposure: In evaluating this question, scientists have examined heavily exposed nonsmokers, specifically, the most readily available data base—nonsmoking women married to smokers. Despite the denials of the tobacco industry and a few independent commentators, the overwhelming number of published "spouse studies" indicate that these high risk women have an increased risk of lung cancer. Admittedly, it is a relatively small increased risk compared to direct smoking. Twenty-four of 30 studies evaluated by EPA found an increased risk, although not all were statistically significant. (The much publicized criticism of the EPA panel using a 90 percent confidence level as opposed to a 95 percent level is a statistical red herring. Any qualified statistician looking at the published data will agree that the findings of a slightly increased lung cancer risk in nonsmoking women did not occur by chance.) The industry argues, in desperation, that a late 1992 study was omitted, thus biasing the EPA conclusion. Actually, the study in question was published after the cut off date and, ironically, would have provided only more support for the EPA findings. The authors noted: "Ours and other recent studies suggest a small but consistent increased risk of lung cancer from passive smoking."

Smoke Is a Carcinogen

Perhaps the most objective evaluation of the cancer risk of passive smoking comes from Sir Richard Doll of Oxford University, who is not specifically known as an anti-smoking activist and is highly regarded by many epidemiologists as the current "dean" of our medical discipline. When I asked him for his assessment on ETS, he wrote "The [World Health Organization] agreed some six or seven years before the EPA that environmental tobacco smoke must be accepted as a human carcinogen. There is a real problem estimating the quantitative effect of environmental tobacco smoke. [But] the suggestion that environmental tobacco smoke is not a human carcinogen can be dismissed as devoid of scientific basis."

As to the non-cancer risks, including asthma and other respiratory distress incurred by nonsmokers, particularly children, the evidence is overwhelming and unequivocal. Children of smokers have higher rates of illness and more school absenteeism. The vast majority of childhood middle ear infections are caused by parental smoking. Staggering health care costs result from the hospitalizations and surgeries (the most common pediatric type) that these infections necessitate. Interestingly, the tobacco industry has not even attempted to deny these data. Philip Morris spokesman Steve Parish agrees that people "should not blow smoke in the face of children. People should use some common sense."

> *"Children of smokers have higher rates of illness and more school absenteeism."*

What should we do? In a January 1993 speech, Michael A. Miles, Chairman of Philip Morris (maker of Marlboros and other tobacco products) likened the ETS "scare" to unfounded panics about cancer-inducing effects of Alar, dioxin and chlorine. Similarly, John Berry, legal counsel for the Council for Burley Tobacco, a party to the lawsuit against EPA, charged "The EPA destroyed the town of Times Beach, Missouri with exaggerated scare tactics on dioxin. If the court does not act in our favor, communities throughout Kentucky . . . will also be destroyed by a government agency that has, quite simply, run amok."

But their analogies comparing trace levels of environmental chemical exposures to ETS fail. The risks of Alar and chlorine in food and water and dioxin in soil are purely hypothetical, based on data from limited animal studies. The cancer risks of ETS, however small, are real. The data are based on human observations.

Who Decides?

Clearly, the health risks of ETS are dose-related. People who live daily in an environment of cigarette smoke are the ones most at risk. Ironically, then, the most risk exists where regulators have no control—in the home. (Increasingly, judges in divorce settlements are taking parental smoking habits into account when assigning custody.) But, other areas of high dose exposure could be the work place, schools, daycare centers, air and ground conveyances and basically anywhere people may be exposed daily over many years. But how much ETS is too much to tolerate, and who decides? This—*not* the question of whether ETS causes human cancer—is the true area of controversy and debate.

The lifetime risk that a nonsmoking woman married to a smoker will develop lung cancer from ETS is estimated to be 1 in 500, as compared to a chance of about 1 in 10 of developing lung cancer from active smoking. But given that the risks of active smoking are so astronomically high compared to other life risks, it is inappropriate to compare passive smoking with the active form. It is better to compare ETS risk with other known human environmental cancer risks, for example, asbestos.

It is possible to argue that we should not tolerate any level of a carcinogen and that, to avoid cancer risk, we should ban smoking in all public places. On the other hand, it is the dose that makes the poison—and transient exposures (like in a fast food restaurant) might thus be irrelevant to lung cancer causation, but not necessarily irrelevant to the causation and exacerbation of acute respiratory distress. Exposures to ETS, however, are cumulative and omnipresent for many of us. The levels of ETS in our lives today far exceed legally tolerated levels of other known human carcinogens—like asbestos—in our highly regulated society.

The question no longer is whether ETS causes lung cancer—it does. The question for the society which takes a regulatory exorcist approach to trace levels of *hypothetical carcinogens* is: At what level will we tolerate a *known human carcinogen?*

Exposure to Secondhand Smoke Is Widespread

by James L. Pirkle et al.

About the author: *James L. Pirkle is the assistant director for science in the Division of Environmental Health Laboratory Sciences at the National Center for Environmental Health of the U.S. Centers for Disease Control and Prevention in Atlanta, Georgia.*

Exposure to environmental tobacco smoke (ETS) [or secondhand smoke] has been associated with acute and chronic health effects among nonsmokers. These effects include lung cancer, asthma, increased incidence of respiratory infections, decreased pulmonary function, and cardiovascular disease. Exposure to ETS may occur in the home, in the workplace, in social settings, and in public places. Data on the extent of exposure to ETS in the US population provide prevalence information for risk assessment and public health prevention strategies, identify population subgroups at increased risk for exposure to ETS, and provide baseline exposure levels that can be compared with future US population levels to evaluate the effectiveness of interventions aimed at reducing ETS exposure. Nevertheless, data are scarce with which to estimate the prevalence of ETS exposure in the US population and in population subgroups, such as children.

In the first phase of the Third National Health and Nutrition Examination Survey (NHANES III), examination and interview data were collected from October 25, 1988, to October 21, 1991, for a representative sample of the civilian, noninstitutionalized US population. The NHANES III included questions on tobacco use and on exposure to ETS at home and at work, as well as measurements of serum cotinine levels. [The human body creates cotinine as a by-product of nicotine.] Cotinine measurements in serum, urine, and saliva are commonly used as a measure of exposure to tobacco smoke. Cotinine is the major metabolite of nicotine and has a half-life of about 16 to 20 hours. Serum cotinine level reflects exposure to nicotine largely from the previous 1 to 2 days. . . .

From James L. Pirkle, Katherine M. Flegal, John T. Bernert, Debra J. Brody, Ruth A. Etzel, Kurt R. Maurer, "Exposure of the U.S. Population to Environmental Tobacco Smoke," *JAMA*, April 24, 1996.

This study assessed the extent of exposure to ETS in the US population. Data from NHANES III were analyzed to estimate the prevalence of reported ETS exposure at home and at work and to describe the determinants of serum cotinine levels among non-tobacco users in a representative national sample.

Subjects and Methods

Phase 1 of NHANES III was conducted from 1988 to 1991 by the National Center for Health Statistics of the Centers for Disease Control and Prevention, Atlanta, Ga. . . .

The protocol included a home interview followed by a physical examination in a mobile examination center. . . .

Reported Tobacco Use and ETS Exposure

Respondents aged 17 years and older were questioned about tobacco use on 2 separate occasions. As part of an interview conducted in the household, respondents aged 17 years and older, who reported that they had smoked at least 100 cigarettes in their lifetime, were asked whether they currently smoked cigarettes. Respondents were also asked whether they currently used other forms of tobacco (cigars, pipes, snuff, or chewing tobacco). A second, private interview was conducted during the examination in the mobile examination center, which usually occurred 2 to 3 weeks after the household interview. In this interview, all respondents, including those who had not reported any tobacco use in the household interview, were questioned about their use of cigarettes, cigars, pipes, snuff, chewing tobacco, and nicotine gum during the past 5 days. Respondents aged 8 to 16 years were questioned about tobacco use only in the mobile examination center. Respondents younger than 8 years were not asked about tobacco use.

"Exposure to environmental tobacco smoke (ETS) has been associated with acute and chronic health effects among nonsmokers."

Reported exposure to ETS at home and at work was defined on the basis of the following questions. For each household participating in the survey, 1 member of the household was asked whether any of the household members smoked cigarettes in the home, and if so, how many cigarettes per day were smoked in the home. If any household member smoked, then each member of that household was classified as being exposed to ETS at home. Adults aged 17 years and older who reported having a job or business were asked how many hours per day they were close enough to tobacco smoke at work so that they could smell the smoke. No questions were asked about smoking by visitors to the home or about exposure to ETS in other settings, such as at social gatherings or in public places.

During the examination, trained dietary interviewers collected detailed information about dietary intake on the previous day for all participants using the

24-hour recall method, in which the respondent is asked to recall and quantify all items of food and drink ingested on the day before the examination. Information was extracted from the dietary database on the weight (in grams) of potatoes, tomatoes, eggplant, cauliflower, and green peppers, either as separate items or as ingredients in mixed dishes, and on the quantity of iced tea and brewed tea consumed. These foods are those previously reported in at least 1 study to have measurable levels of nicotine.

> *"Of adult non-tobacco users, 37.4% reported exposure to ETS at home or at work."*

During the examination in the mobile examination center, blood samples were drawn for serum cotinine analysis. . . .

Reported Exposure to ETS

The estimated prevalences of reported ETS exposure at home and of reported tobacco use for children and adolescents aged 2 months to 16 years in the US population are given in Table 1. Within each age group, the proportion with reported ETS exposure was slightly higher for females than males. The prevalence of non-tobacco users with ETS exposure was lower among adolescents. For ages 2 months to 11 years, the prevalence of reported ETS exposure at home was 43%.

The estimated prevalences of reported ETS exposure at home or at work and of reported tobacco use are given in Table 2 by age and sex for adults aged 17 years and older in the US population. Of adult non-tobacco users, 37.4% reported exposure to ETS at home or at work, with the percentage of males (43.5%) being somewhat higher than that of females (32.9%). The prevalence of reported ETS exposure among non-tobacco users was 36.9% for non-Hispanic blacks, 37.4% for non-Hispanic whites, and 35.1% for Mexican Americans. Of working adults who were non-tobacco users, 47.7% reported exposure to ETS at home or at work. For non-tobacco users who were exposed to ETS at work, the mean duration of exposure was 4.4 hours. . . .

Of those exposed to smoke in their homes, most had only 1 household member who smoked in the home. Only 4.7% of persons exposed to ETS at home had more than 2 smokers in the household. . . .

Serum Cotinine Levels

Among non-tobacco users, those who reported exposure tended to have higher levels of serum cotinine than did those with no reported exposure. Of persons who reported they were non-tobacco users, 87.9% had detectable levels of cotinine in their serum. Of tobacco users and non-tobacco users considered together, 91.7% had detectable levels of cotinine. . . .

Cotinine levels were higher in persons with reported home ETS exposure than in those with no reported home or work ETS exposure. In working adults, cotinine levels were highest in the home and work exposure group, followed by home exposure only, work exposure only, and no home or work exposure. Among age groups, the serum cotinine levels were similar in the category of no home or work exposure but tended to decline in the home exposure category as age increased. . . .

Exposures to ETS at home and at work were significantly and consistently associated with serum cotinine levels and accounted for most of the explained variance. Some sociodemographic and behavioral variables were also significantly associated with serum cotinine levels. None of the dietary factors was consistently associated with serum cotinine levels across the 3 age groups. Amount of bell peppers consumed was significant for children only, and amount of potatoes consumed was significant for adolescents only. None of the foods was significant for adults. Comparisons of models with and without the dietary variables showed that the group of dietary variables explained less than 2% of the variance of serum cotinine level. . . .

Widespread Exposure

Exposure to ETS has been identified as a health hazard for adults and children. Data from NHANES III (1988–1991) provide the first opportunity to estimate the extent of exposure to ETS in the US population on the basis of questionnaire data and of serum cotinine measurements in a large representative national sample. The questionnaire data from NHANES III showed that 43% of US children are exposed to smoking by household members. Of the adult nontobacco-using population, 37% reported home or work exposure to ETS. Serum

Table 1.—Percentage of Persons with Reported Tobacco Use and Reported Exposure to ETS by Sex and Age for Children and Adolescents Aged 2 Months to 16 Years: United States, 1988–1991*

Sex and Age	Sample Size	Reported No Tobacco Use, %		Reported Tobacco Use,%‡
		No Reported Home ETS Exposure	Reported Home ETS Exposure†	
All				
2 mo-3 y	**3185**	59.2	40.8	. . .
4-11 y	**3011**	56.3	43.6	0.1
12-16 y	**883**	52.4	35.7	11.9
Males				
2 mo-3 y	1547	61.4	38.6	. . .
4-11 y	1493	57.5	42.3	0.2
12-16 y	425	52.3	33.9	13.9
Females				
2 mo-3 y	1638	56.9	43.1	. . .
4-11 y	1518	55.0	45.0	0.1
12-16 y	458	52.5	37.6	9.9

* ETS indicates environmental tobacco smoke. Rows may not add to 100% because of rounding.
† Based on reported smoking in the home by members of the household.
‡ Children younger than 8 years were not asked about use of tobacco products. Tobacco products included cigarettes, cigars, pipes, snuff, chewing tobacco, and nicotine gum.

Table 2.—Percentage of Persons with Reported Tobacco Use and Reported Exposure to ETS by Sex and Age for Adults 17 Years of Age and Older: United States, 1988–1991*

		Reported No Tobacco Use, %				
Sex and Age, y	Sample Size	No Reported Home or Work ETS Exposure	Reported Home ETS Exposure Only	Reported Work ETS Exposure Only	Reported Home and Work ETS Exposure	Reported Tobacco Use, %
All	**9769**	38.8	7.7	12.4	3.1	38.0
Males						
≥17	**4863**	30.8	6.2	14.8	2.8	45.3
17-19	296	26.8	16.1	13.0	6.5	36.7
20-29	917	22.6	7.3	15.2	2.7	52.2
30-39	822	26.2	3.9	17.9	2.3	49.7
40-49	672	24.8	3.7	18.8	2.8	49.9
50-59	524	29.5	4.8	17.7	4.8	43.3
60-69	634	48.3	7.5	9.1	1.2	33.9
≥70	998	62.5	6.8	2.1	0.3	28.4
Females						
≥17	**4906**	46.0	9.2	10.1	3.4	31.3
17-19	308	38.1	16.1	8.8	5.9	31.1
20-29	893	32.7	10.2	14.7	4.7	37.6
30-39	839	41.1	7.3	11.0	4.3	36.4
40-49	644	39.9	9.5	14.0	4.7	32.0
50-59	502	43.4	11.4	11.2	2.5	31.5
60-69	661	62.7	6.1	4.6	0.6	25.8
≥70	1059	76.8	7.4	0.3	0.0	15.5

* ETS indicates environmental tobacco smoke. Tobacco products included cigarettes, cigars, pipes, snuff, chewing tobacco, and nicotine gum.

cotinine measurements showed even more widespread exposure to nicotine in the population. Of persons who were non-tobacco users, 87.9% had detectable levels of cotinine. The most likely source of these detectable levels of cotinine is exposure to ETS. Any contributions of underreporting of smoking status or of dietary nicotine seem to be minimal. Thus, the NHANES III data indicate widespread exposure to ETS in the US population. . . .

Measurements of serum cotinine supported the validity of the reports of ETS exposure in NHANES III. In every age group, those with reported ETS exposure showed higher levels of serum cotinine than those with no reported ETS exposure. Reported exposure was highly significantly associated with serum cotinine levels even after adjusting for age, sociodemographic factors, behavioral variables, and dietary intake. A high percentage of the variance in serum cotinine levels among non-tobacco users was explained by reported ETS exposure.

Most of the non-tobacco-using population, including those who reported no exposure to ETS at work or from smoking by household members, had detectable levels of serum cotinine, indicating even more widespread exposure to nicotine than reflected by the questionnaire data. . . .

The most likely source of the widespread nicotine exposure reflected in serum cotinine levels is ETS exposure from reported home and work exposures as well as exposures to ETS not captured by the questions on home and work exposure. The questionnaire data did not address all possible sources of ETS exposure. Questions were asked about household members who smoked in the home, but not about smoking by guests and visitors to the household. No questions were asked about exposure to ETS in public places, in social settings, during transportation, or in other nonwork, nonhome locations, and no questions were asked about recent ETS exposure in general. In addition, respondents may not be aware of some ETS exposure that may have occurred at home or work. . . .

ETS Exposure at Home and Work

The prevalence of reported exposure to ETS at home was higher among children than among adult non-tobacco users, confirming the importance of smoking in the home in determining the extent to which children involuntarily inhale the tobacco smoke of others. More than 40% of children aged 4 to 11 years reported home ETS exposure. This finding is similar to what has been reported among children in other communities in the United States. For example, the 1988 National Health Interview Survey data showed that 42.5% of children aged 5 years and younger were exposed to a smoker in their households. . . .

More than 23% of the US population of adults aged 17 years and older reported home or work ETS exposure. Among adult non-tobacco users, the prevalence of reported exposure to ETS at work was greater than that of the prevalence of reported exposure to ETS at home. In the California Activity Pattern Survey (1987–1988), researchers found that time spent at work was highly correlated with ETS exposure. Additional studies have indicated that the workplace is a major source of ETS exposure, especially among nonsmokers who are not exposed at home. In our study, the prevalence of reported exposure at work was higher than the prevalence of reported exposure at home. Serum cotinine levels were higher in those with reported ETS exposure at home only than in those with reported ETS exposure at work only. The highest cotinine levels among non-tobacco users were found in those who reported home and work exposure. . . .

> *"Cotinine levels were higher in persons with reported home ETS exposure."*

Public Health Implications

The NHANES III data indicate widespread exposure to ETS in the population. Exposure to ETS has been associated with increased risk for lung cancer and cardiovascular disease among adults and with impaired lung function and respiratory problems among children. Many of these studies are based on reported exposure rather than on measured serum cotinine levels. The NHANES III data suggest that there may be considerable exposure even within the comparison groups in studies of the effects of ETS. If so, these studies may underestimate risk from ETS exposure.

These cotinine levels reflect the amount of exposure to tobacco smoke and its toxic constituents. Further research is needed to define better the degree of health risk associated with specific levels of serum cotinine.

Chapter 2

Is the Tobacco Industry to Blame for Leading People to Smoke?

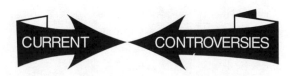

Chapter Preface

In 1965, the U.S. Congress passed the Federal Cigarette Labeling and Advertising Act. This law required cigarette companies to place the following warning on all cigarette packages:

> CAUTION: CIGARETTE SMOKING MAY BE HAZARDOUS TO YOUR HEALTH.

The law was passed as a result of the historic 1964 surgeon general's report that linked smoking to lung cancer and other diseases. This report and the relatively minor warning were the first salvos in the fight between the tobacco industry and advocates of increased government regulation of tobacco.

Those who support government regulation of tobacco argue that the tobacco industry is more concerned about profit than the public's health. The industry is widely criticized for knowingly producing a harmful product and encouraging its consumption through advertising and promotion. Terry A. Rustin, an assistant professor at the University of Texas Medical School, expresses the view held by many people when he states, "Tobacco companies are selling death and disease and making huge profits." Rustin and others argue that the tobacco companies' indifference toward the public's health makes increased regulation of tobacco advertising and sales necessary.

However, regulation opponents maintain that the industry has been unfairly blamed for the harms caused by smoking. They contend that tobacco companies do not force people to smoke; rather, people choose to smoke. As conservative columnist Mona Charen writes, "People are well-informed about the dangers of smoking and fully capable of stopping but smoke anyway." Charen, along with other conservatives and business supporters, insists that since people are free to make their own decisions about whether or not to smoke, increased government regulation of the industry is not justified as a means of protecting the public from the harmful effects of smoking.

Due to public concern about the health consequences of smoking, the tobacco industry has fallen under intense scrutiny. In the following chapters, authors debate whether the industry intentionally lures people to smoking by means of advertising and whether it addicts smokers to cigarettes by manipulating the nicotine levels in tobacco.

Tobacco Ads Deceive People into Smoking

by Terry A. Rustin

About the author: *Terry A. Rustin is an assistant professor at the University of Texas Medical School in Houston.*

The tobacco companies have been analyzing your fantasies, and they want you to know that, whatever your fantasy, cigarettes should be a part of it. Whether you want to be strong or sexy, independent or gregarious, Philip Morris, RJR Nabisco, Lorillard and American Brands are eager to help you.

The tobacco companies promote specific images and lifestyles to help convince current smokers to switch brands, former smokers to resume their addiction and young people to begin smoking for the first time. Advertisements over the years have featured sports heroes, movie stars, doctors, babies, horses and cowboys, among others, to promote cigarettes to different demographic groups.

Five of the most popular brands—and most heavily promoted—are Philip Morris' Marlboro and Virginia Slims, RJR Nabisco's Camel, Lorillard's Newport and American Brands' Carlton. They have raised product promotion to an art form.

Marketing Camels to Kids

Camels, the first cigarette produced by the R.J. Reynolds family, hit the market in 1913. They were inexpensive, uniform, flavorful and convenient. They contained "Turkish and domestic tobaccos" and carried a picture of a camel on the desert with the pyramids in the background. Heavily promoted using posters and handbills, Camels took advantage of America's fascination with exotic places and were marketed as the cigarette for the tough, uncompromising man. By 1919, Camels controlled 38 percent of the cigarette market.

From their introduction until 1987, Camels were promoted as a man's cigarette. In 1987, however, on the occasion of the 75th anniversary of their introduction, and in response to sagging market share, R.J. Reynolds introduced a

Terry A. Rustin, "Death and Disease for Sale." Reprinted with permission from *Priorities* (Winter 1993), a publication of the American Council on Science and Health, 1995 Broadway, 2nd Floor, New York, NY 10023-5860.

bold new advertising campaign using a cartoon camel as its motif. Known as "Old Joe" (the name of the circus camel that served as a model for the original Camel package), this cartoon character is featured in dozens of ads in magazines and on billboards engaged in typical dromedary activities—astride a motorcycle in full leathers, water skiing, lounging outside a Las Vegas nightclub and dragging a young woman up the beach by her hair. Joe Camel and his friends in "The Hard Pack" are oh-so-cool as they live out the ideal spring break sophomoric fantasy. Young smokers can partake in the fantasy by purchasing clothing, mugs, Swiss army knives, hats and other merchandise with Camel cash, coupons inserted into cigarette packs.

A Great Success

Smokin' Joe has been a great success. According to a study published in the *Journal of the American Medical Association* (*JAMA*), Joe is recognized by 91.3 percent of 6-year-olds and 31 percent of 3-year-olds. In 1987, according to *JAMA*, Camels were the preferred cigarette of only 0.5 percent of children under 19; by 1991, 32.8 percent of them preferred Camels. Since the introduction of Joe Camel, teen smoking has increased by ten percent, according to the *Tobacco and Youth Reporter*. Furthermore, the *New York Times* (7/29/92) reported that while the market share of most full-priced cigarette brands has been falling, Camel market share climbed to 4.5 percent.

> *"The tobacco companies promote specific images and lifestyles."*

But tobacco companies insist they do not advertise to children. Philip Morris has even taken out magazine ads telling teens that they are too young to make the decision to smoke, and that smoking is only for adults. What better way to get adolescents to smoke! The ads never mention the real reasons not to smoke: lung cancer, emphysema, stroke, heart disease, *etc*.

Regardless of what the tobacco companies say, their advertisements are sufficiently attractive to children to convince thousands of them to start smoking every year. Today, more teenage girls than boys start smoking. If the trend continues, by the year 2000, there will be more female than male smokers for the first time in history. The trend is already evident in cancer mortality statistics—lung cancer has recently surpassed breast cancer as the leading cancer killer in women.

Marlboro: Determination and Adventure

Philip Morris' premier product, Marlboro, was originally a woman's cigarette (complete with a red filter to hide lipstick marks) with cute babies in its advertisements. In 1954, Philip Morris devised a new image for Marlboro, that looks down on us today from thousands of billboards—the steely eyes and gritty determination of the Marlboro Man. One of those original Marlboro cowboys was

Wayne McLaren, who died at age 51 of lung cancer in 1992.

Today, Marlboro is the most popular brand of cigarette in the U.S., holding 23 percent of the cigarette market. Around the world, Marlboro is the cigarette of fearless, confident women and men—or at least, women and men who can imagine themselves fearless and confident while they smoke a Marlboro.

Today, Philip Morris is again repositioning Marlboro, this time as a cigarette for adventurous young people. The current Marlboro campaign—estimated to be costing the company $200 million—offers smokers of Marlboro an opportunity to be part of the "Marlboro Adventure Team." A ten-page advertisement featured in *Rolling Stone* and other popular magazines showed typical Marlboro smokers white-river rafting, riding a motorcycle through the desert and challenging the outback in a sporty truck. Older smokers may find contentment imagining themselves relaxing beside a campfire, but younger ones want thrills and challenges. Now Marlboro offers both visions as part of its updated image. The aging Marlboro smoker (who remembers the Marlboro TV ads) will see the Marlboro cowboy in *Time*, *Newsweek* and *Sports Illustrated*; the younger smoker will see the Adventure Team in youth-oriented publications.

From a business perspective, this approach makes good sense. The loyal Marlboro smoker, a good customer for 20 or 30 or more years, will soon die from lung cancer, emphysema or heart disease. The tobacco companies lose 5,000 of their best customers every day and must replace them. By appealing to more intrepid and more reckless young people, Marlboro hopes to attract another generation of smokers.

Newport Finds a Niche Market

Lorillard has targeted its menthol cigarette, Newport, at African-American men and women. In cities across the country, Newport ads fill billboards in areas where African-Americans live. They appear prominently in the African-American oriented magazines and newspapers. These ads show people enjoying sports, jazz music and each other's company. "Alive with pleasure," the Newport slogan, gives a strong message that counters the Surgeon General's warnings. Given that African-Americans already have higher death rates from heart disease, stroke and cancer than whites, "Killed for pleasure" would be more accurate.

> *"Their advertisements are sufficiently attractive to children to convince thousands of them to start smoking every year."*

Many Newport ads concentrate on relationships. One shows a young African-American couple on a park bench. His head rests on her lap as she drops popcorn into his mouth. They are having a wonderful relaxing time. There are no cigarettes in the ad at all. In an age where the deterioration of family life is a paramount issue in the African-American community, this ad suggests that Newport will somehow keep this couple together and happy.

Newport adds menthol to its tobacco. The ads for Newport, Salem, Kool and Doral suggest that menthol adds a "fresh taste." Actually, menthol is an anaesthetic that partially numbs the throat so that smokers will not feel the burn as poisonous smoke scorches their throats. The menthol simply makes it easier for the addicted smoker to smoke more.

Courting the Anorectic Woman

Philip Morris has profited from women's desire to be thin with Virginia Slims. In order to convince women that they should start smoking, relapse to smoking or change brands, the tobacco companies portray women smokers as young, independent, stylish, healthy and thin—*extremely* thin. Some of the ads even distort images of the female models, making them even taller and slimmer than they actually are. The product names emphasize thinness: Virginia Slims, SuperSlims and the new product, Saratoga Lights New Slim 100s. These messages help keep women addicted to tobacco. The ads glamorize an unhealthy body image and emphasize that smoking is the easiest way to stay thin.

"The tobacco companies lose 5,000 of their best customers every day and must replace them."

These ads distort scientific data. Research published in the *New England Journal of Medicine* documents that regular smoking increases a person's metabolic rate by about ten percent. When people stop smoking but fail to change their eating or exercise habits, they will gain weight, but according to Ellen Gritz, Ph.D., a UCLA psychologist, the gain is usually about five pounds. For an overly weight conscious woman, five pounds is not only unacceptable in itself, it heralds even greater weight gain. She retreats back to her old friend, cigarettes.

These cigarette ads also promise women independence and power. "You've come a long way, baby," is the rather demeaning slogan that heralds women's entrance into the business world. It also invites women into the world of smoking addiction, a world where independence is exchanged for a life threatening dependence on nicotine.

Marketing to the Health Conscious

Carlton, made by American Brands, focuses its ads on claims that "Carlton is lowest" in tar and nicotine delivery. The Surgeon General calls such statements "implied health claims." The ads aren't quite saying, "Carltons are safe cigarettes," but that is certainly the intended message. To the smoker who wishes to quit for health reasons but is having difficulty, the "lowest" message gives him or her a psychologically pleasing alternative to giving up cigarettes altogether. The truth is that there is no scientific evidence that any one brand of cigarette is safer than another, regardless of the measured tar and nicotine delivery. All cigarettes cause heart disease, cancer and emphysema at about the same rate.

It is true that "Carlton is lowest" in tar and nicotine delivery, but only under the conditions of Federal Trade Commission tests, in which a machine holds the test cigarette by its tip and smokes it in a standardized fashion. The Carlton cigarette has tiny holes in the paper that allow air into the smoke stream, cooling the tars and precipitating them on the filter. However, under actual smoking conditions, smokers tend to cover up the holes with their fingers, defeating the low tar strategy. The smoker really gets a full dose of carcinogens.

Selling Death and Disease for Profit

These campaigns by the tobacco companies exploit our fears, appeal to our fantasies and fool our children. Tobacco companies are selling death and disease and making huge profits. As long as Joe Camel is allowed to leer at us from thousands of billboards, and Virginia Slims women tempt us from the pages of popular magazines, we and our children will continue to be influenced in favor of smoking. Only by either banning tobacco promotions of all kinds, or by requiring honest counteradvertising, will we effectively rebut these insidious messages.

Tobacco Ads Target Children

by *America*

About the author: America *is a weekly Catholic magazine of opinion on social, political, and religious issues.*

"Got a light?" Older Americans might associate this question with sophisticated adults in a movie from the 1940's or 1950's. Nowadays, however, it is frequently being asked by children under 18. Health officials estimate that each day 3,000 children start smoking, most of them between the ages of 10 and 18; they account for 90 percent of all new smokers. A third will die of smoking-related diseases.

New Regulations

In an effort to curb tobacco use among youth, the Department of Health and Human Services issued regulations in January 1996, aimed at enforcing the ban on selling tobacco to anyone under 18 by penalizing states that do not monitor tobacco sales in stores. But the very fact that the tobacco industry supports the new regulations suggests they may lack teeth. Health advocates and anti-smoking groups contend that far more is needed, notably proposals made by the Food and Drug Administration in July 1995. At that time the F.D.A. urged that nicotine be classified as an addictive drug, that cigarette vending machines be banned (a major source of tobacco for the underaged) and that advertising aimed at youth be restricted.

In August President Clinton, to his credit, supported the F.D.A. proposals and expressed his hope that smoking by children and teen-agers could be reduced by 50 percent within seven years after the proposals receive congressional approval. But the F.D.A.'s desire to classify nicotine as an addictive drug is sure to be fiercely resisted by the tobacco industry, as will restrictions on advertising. Resistance can also be expected from members of Congress representing tobacco growing states, as well as from those who receive substantial contributions from the industry. In the first half of 1995, the industry donated $1.5 million to the Republican Party treasury, a 400 percent increase over the previous year's contribution in the same period.

Targeting Youth

Especially disturbing to child health advocates is advertising that targets youth. A study described in the *Journal of the American Medical Association* (12/11/91) noted that among children of kindergarten age, R.J. Reynolds's cartoon character, Joe Camel, is as familiar as the Mickey Mouse logo of the Disney television channel. Two other studies released in October and November of 1995—one reported in the *Journal of the National Cancer Institute*, the other in *Health Psychology*—found that children receptive to advertising are two to four times as likely to begin smoking as those who are not and that there is a correlation between promotional campaigns with free T-shirts and the like and smoking among children aged 14 to 17.

The industry denies targeting people under 21 and claims that its advertising goal is simply to promote brand switching and brand loyalty. But it is well aware that children and teens do not have the experience and information to weigh the dangers of smoking. That is why they represent what one anti-smoking advocate, Representative Henry A. Waxman, Democrat of California, has called a tobacco advertiser's dream. An internal R.J. Reynolds memo obtained and described by the *Washington Post* (10/14/95) shows that as early as 1973 the youth market was being kept in careful focus. The memo outlines a strategy for attracting what it calls "learning smokers." Scott Ballin, chairman of the Coalition on Smoking OR Health—composed of the American Cancer Society, the American Lung Association and the American Heart Association—described the memo as clear evidence of youth targeting.

> *"Children receptive to advertising are two to four times as likely to begin smoking as those who are not."*

Pregnant teens and young women are at particular risk because of the danger to their unborn children. Smoking during pregnancy is linked with increased risk of infant mortality and low birth weight. William J. Cox, executive director of the Catholic Health Association, described this aspect of the situation as a pro-life matter: "The pro-life community is committed to protecting not only the life of the unborn child, but its health as well."

Mr. Cox also noted that young women in their teens represent the largest group of new smokers. This may be the result, at least in part, of the barrage of advertising specifically directed toward them since the late 1960's. Ad campaigns like that of Philip Morris for its highly successful Virginia Slims brand, using the slogan "You've Come a Long Way, Baby," have been associated with sudden increases in smoking by girls 11 to 17 years old. The appeal of such ads, with their use of magic words like "slim," is especially strong for those who may be self-conscious about their weight.

For these and other young women who become addicted and continue smoking, the price in terms of mortality is high. As a direct result of increased tobacco use, lung cancer now surpasses breast cancer as the number one cause of cancer deaths among women. The tobacco industry is well aware of facts like these but places concern for profit above considerations of public health. After all, if children and teen-agers did not begin smoking, the industry's sales in this country would shrivel up—and more Americans would not have their lives cut short. A telling cartoon in the *Philadelphia Inquirer* shows an industry representative saying: "Hardly anyone over 21 starts smoking. We don't *want* to target your kids. We have no choice." In the final panel of the cartoon we see the representative standing by a crib; in it, a baby reaches up toward toys suspended from a mobile above in the shape of cigarette packs and, yes, the head of Joc Camel.

Tobacco Companies Control Nicotine Levels in Cigarettes to Addict Smokers

by David A. Kessler

About the author: *David A. Kessler is the commissioner of food and drugs for the U.S. Food and Drug Administration, the government agency that conducts research and develops standards on the safety of food, drugs, and health-related products.*

Editor's note: The following was excerpted from testimony delivered before the U.S. House of Representatives Subcommittee on Health and the Environment on June 21, 1994.

In my last appearance before this subcommittee on March 25, 1994, . . . I reviewed the evidence that supports the scientific consensus that nicotine is addictive. I also reviewed the evidence we had at that time on the ability of the tobacco industry to control nicotine levels, including numerous industry patents for technologies to manipulate and control nicotine content. I described activities of the cigarette industry that resemble those of pharmaceutical manufacturers. I presented information that raised the question of whether tobaccos were blended to manipulate and control nicotine levels. And I provided data showing that over the last decade, nicotine levels have not dropped in parallel with tar levels—in fact, they have risen.

We have continued to focus our analysis and investigation on the physiological and pharmacological effects of nicotine and on the degree to which cigarette companies manipulate and control the level of nicotine in their products.

The information that I presented about industry control and manipulation of nicotine the last time I testified before you was suggestive. Today I am going to

From David A. Kessler's "Statement on the Control and Manipulation of Nicotine in Cigarettes" to the House Committee on Energy and Commerce, Subcommittee on Health and Environment, June 21, 1994.

provide you with actual instances of control and manipulation of nicotine by some in the tobacco industry that have been uncovered through painstaking investigational work.

We have discovered that manipulation of nicotine has been carried out by some even before tobacco seeds were planted in the fields. We have discovered other forms of manipulation that occur later, in the design and manufacture of cigarettes.

Today I want to discuss two examples of nicotine manipulation in some detail. First, we have discovered the deliberate *genetic* manipulation of the nicotine content in a tobacco plant. It is the story of how an American tobacco company spent more than a decade quietly developing a high-nicotine tobacco plant, growing it in Central and South America, and using it in American cigarettes. Second, I will discuss how chemical compounds are added to cigarettes to manipulate nicotine delivery.

The Story of Y-1

The project I am going to tell you about led to development of a tobacco plant code-named "Y-1." It has been an enormous task to piece together the picture of Y-1. Confidentiality agreements have made getting the facts very difficult.

The story begins in Portuguese with our discovery of a Brazilian patent for a new variety of a flue-cured tobacco plant. One sentence of its English translation caught our eye. "The nicotine content of the leaf of this variety is usually higher than approximately 6% by weight . . . which is significantly higher than any normal variety of tobacco grown commercially."

Prior to our discovery of the patent, J.W. Johnson, the chief executive officer of R.J. Reynolds Tobacco Company, had told us that "flue-cured tobacco naturally contains 2.5 to 3.5 percent nicotine." Thus, this new specially bred plant would contain approximately twice the nicotine that naturally occurs in flue-cured tobacco.

"Manipulation of nicotine has been carried out by some even before tobacco seeds were planted in the fields."

The holder of the Brazilian Y-1 patent was Brown & Williamson Tobacco Corporation, maker of such cigarettes as Kool, Viceroy, Richland, Barclay, and Raleigh.

An Interesting Discovery

Let me tell you why this discovery interested us. Industry representatives have repeatedly stated for the public record that they do not manipulate nicotine levels in cigarettes. The plant described in this patent represents a dramatic attempt to manipulate nicotine.

Moreover, when we asked company officials whether plants were bred specifically for higher nicotine content, we were told that this was not feasible. We were told that tobacco growers and cigarette manufacturers have an agreement that the nicotine level of new varieties of tobacco grown in the United States can vary only slightly from the levels of standard varieties. Under this agreement, a new high-nicotine tobacco plant that varied more than slightly from the standard variety could not be commercially grown by farmers in the United States.

Nevertheless, we learned that interest in developing a high-nicotine tobacco plant dates back to at least the mid-1970's. In 1977, Dr. James F. Chaplin, then of both the USDA [United States Department of Agriculture] and North Carolina State University, stated:

> manufacturers have means of reducing tars but most of the methods reduce nicotine and other constituents at the same time. Therefore it may be desirable to develop levels constant or to develop lines higher in nicotine so that when the tar and nicotine are reduced there will still be enough nicotine left to satisfy the smoker.

In fact, Dr. Chaplin had been working on genetically breeding tobacco plants with varying nicotine levels. In a 1977 paper, Dr. Chaplin indicated that tobacco could be bred to increase nicotine levels, specifically by cross breeding commercial varieties of tobacco with *Nicotiana rustica*. *N. rustica* is a wild variety, very high in nicotine, but not used commercially in cigarettes because it is considered too harsh. . . .

Breeding the New Variety of Tobacco

Over the next several years Dr. Chaplin continued his efforts to breed a tobacco plant with a higher nicotine level. During that time, an employee of a Brown & Williamson–affiliated company asked Dr. Chaplin for some of his seeds. Some of Dr. Chaplin's original plant varieties were used as a basis for Brown & Williamson's work. From what we can gather, there was no formal release of this high-nicotine tobacco variety for private use. In the early 1980's, Brown & Williamson grew a number of different plant lines on its experimental farm in Wilson, North Carolina, selecting those that had the best agronomic characteristics.

In 1983, Brown & Williamson contracted with DNA Plant Technology to work on tobacco breeding. Much of the developmental work on Y-1 took place in the laboratories, greenhouses, and fields owned by DNA Plant Technology. After he retired from USDA, in 1986, Brown & Williamson also hired Dr. Chaplin as a consultant to work on Y-1 and other projects.

"What was accomplished was the development of a tobacco plant with a high-nicotine content."

The high-nicotine tobacco variety Y-1 was developed by a combination of conventional and advanced genetic breeding techniques. . . .

What was accomplished was the development of a tobacco plant with a high-nicotine content—about 6 percent—that grew well and could be used commercially. . . .

On Friday June 17, 1994, . . . Brown & Williamson told FDA that, in fact, three and a half to four million pounds of Y-1 tobacco are currently being stored in company warehouses in the United States. More significantly, Brown & Williamson revealed that Y-1 had, in fact, been commercialized.

These brands of cigarettes—Viceroy King Size, Viceroy Lights King Size, Richland King Size, Richland Lights King Size, and Raleigh Lights King Size—were manufactured and distributed nationally in 1993 with a tobacco blend that contains approximately 10 percent of this genetically-bred high-nicotine tobacco called Y-1.

The Chemical Manipulation of Nicotine

In April 1994, the six major American cigarette companies released a list of 599 ingredients added to tobacco. Nicotine is not one of the additives listed. But a number of chemicals on that list increase the amount of nicotine that is delivered to the smoker.

Around the time the list was made public, a great deal of interest was directed toward substances on the list that sounded particularly toxic. Among those frequently mentioned was ammonia. Many people may have wondered why the cigarette industry would add ammonia to tobacco. In fact, there are many uses of ammonia. Our investigations have revealed an important one.

Let me refer to a major American tobacco company's 1991 handbook on leaf blending and product development. The handbook describes two ways that ammonia can be used in cigarette manufacture. One way is to interact with sugars in the tobacco. But it is the second way, the effect of ammonia and related compounds on the delivery of nicotine to the smoker, that is most striking. Let me quote from that handbook: "[The ammonia in the cigarette smoke] can liberate free nicotine from the blend, which is associated with increases in impact and 'satisfaction' reported by smokers.". . . It is important to emphasize here that most of the nicotine in the average American cigarette is in the bound form. By that I mean it is not going to readily make its way to the smoker. . . . Only a fraction of the nicotine in the tobacco gets inhaled by the smoker. The handbook indicates that this ammonia technology enables more nicotine to be delivered to the smoker than if the ammonia technology is not employed. . . . How much additional nicotine does this technology impart? It is our understanding, based on smoke analysis described in the company handbook, that an experimental cigarette made of reconstituted tobacco treated with ammonia has almost double the nicotine transfer efficiency of tobacco.

> *"An experimental cigarette . . . treated with ammonia has almost double the nicotine transfer efficiency of [standard] tobacco."*

Many Companies Use Ammonia

How widespread is ammonia use in the industry? The company handbook states that many U.S. tobacco companies use ammonia technologies. Until we have access to similar documents from other companies, we will not know whether other companies use it directly to affect nicotine levels.

To determine how well nicotine content is controlled in cigarettes, FDA laboratories compared the content uniformity of drugs in either tablets or capsules to the content uniformity of nicotine in cigarettes. What is striking is how little the nicotine content varies from cigarette to cigarette, suggesting tight and precise control of the amount of nicotine in cigarettes. In fact, the nicotine content uniformity of the cigarettes tested meets drug content uniformity standards set by the U.S. Pharmacopeia.

"Some in the industry have identified target levels of nicotine necessary to satisfy smokers' desire for nicotine."

I have presented information on the control and manipulation of nicotine because I believe it raises certain important questions—questions that are even more important in light of the repeated assertions of the cigarette industry that it does not control or manipulate nicotine. Why spend a decade developing through genetic breeding a high-nicotine tobacco and adding that tobacco to cigarettes if you are not interested in controlling and manipulating nicotine? Why focus on the enhanced delivery of free nicotine to the smoker by chemical manipulation if you are not interested in controlling and manipulating nicotine?

The Goals of Control and Manipulation

Why is there such interest in controlling and manipulating nicotine in cigarettes? Senior industry officials are aware that nicotine is the critical ingredient in cigarettes. Some in the industry have identified target levels of nicotine necessary to satisfy smokers' desire for nicotine. And the industry has undertaken research into nicotine's physiologic and pharmacologic effects.

Let me give you one example of how a company has identified specific levels of nicotine necessary to satisfy smokers and focused on how to achieve those levels. A company document describes consumer preference testing on "impact," which according to the company correlates with nicotine. The document states that impact is a "high priority" attribute of cigarettes and is: ". . . controllable to relatively fine tolerances by product development/product intervention . . . (by manipulating nicotine in blend/smoke. . .)."

This document goes on to describe an elaborate model for establishing the minimum and maximum nicotine levels tolerated by consumers. . . . It is thus clear that at least one major cigarette manufacturer is aware of the need to target nicotine delivery to levels necessary to satisfy smokers. In fact, as tobacco flavor specialist A.N. Hertz has written, one of the most important goals of cigarette design is to "ensure high satisfaction from an adequate level of nicotine per puff," and that even cigarettes with reduced levels of nicotine and tar must have this property.

A Fine Drug

Publicly available information, including recently released documents, reveals much about the industry's knowledge of the drug-like effects of nicotine. . . .

Let me quote some of the recently reported statements of officials from one company that reveal a recognition of nicotine's drug-like effects:

> Nicotine is not only a very fine drug, but the techniques of administration by smoking has considerable psychological advantages.

> . . . nicotine is a very remarkable, beneficent drug that both helps the body to resist external stress and also can, as a result, show a pronounced tranquilizing effect.

These statements were apparently made by Sir Charles Ellis, a member of the Royal Society of London, who served as science advisor to the board of British American Tobacco Company. . . . Two of his recently reported statements are particularly striking. One statement was made in 1962: "Smoking is a habit of addiction."

But perhaps the most striking statement attributed to him is one from a meeting of company scientists in 1967 [recorded in a British American Tobacco Company research chronology]: "Sir Charles Ellis states that BATCO is in the nicotine rather than the tobacco industry."

These statements are echoed by those made in an internal company document by another senior scientist at a British tobacco company:

> There is now no doubt that nicotine plays a large part in the action of smoking for many smokers. It may be useful, therefore, to look at the tobacco industry as if for a large part its business is the administration of nicotine (in the clinical sense).

These statements are consistent with the quotes from William L. Dunn, an official of Philip Morris:

> Think of the cigarette pack as a storage container for a day's supply of nicotine.

> Think of the cigarette as a dispenser for a dose unit of nicotine.

> Think of a puff of smoke as the vehicle for nicotine.

> Smoke is beyond question the most optimized vehicle of nicotine . . .

The Addictive Nature of Nicotine

Other scientists are quoted in a May 30, 1963 paper that is reported to have been produced for Brown & Williamson's sister company, the British American

Tobacco Company, and labeled "Confidential: A Tentative Hypothesis on Nicotine Addiction." As reported, it contains a number of statements regarding the powerful effect of nicotine on the body:

> Chronic intake of nicotine tends to restore the normal physiological functioning of the endocrine system, so that ever-increasing dose levels of nicotine are necessary to maintain the desired action. Unlike other dopings, such as morphine, the demand for increasing dose levels is relatively slow for nicotine.

Other statements reportedly made in this paper speak directly to the addictive nature of nicotine. The report goes on to describe what happens when a chronic smoker is denied nicotine: "A body left in this unbalanced state craves for renewed drug intake in order to restore the physiological equilibrium. This unconscious desire explains the addiction of the individual to nicotine."

Selling an Addictive Drug

The information that we have presented today has been the result of painstaking investigation. We now know that a tobacco company commercially developed a tobacco plant with twice the nicotine content of standard tobacco, that several million pounds of this high-nicotine tobacco are currently stored in warehouses, and that this tobacco was put into cigarettes that have been sold nationwide. We now know that several tobacco companies add ammonia compounds to cigarettes, and that one company's documents confirm that one of the intended purposes of this practice is to manipulate nicotine delivery to the smoker. And we now know that some in the industry have identified target ranges of nicotine delivery. These findings lay to rest any notion that there is no manipulation and control of nicotine undertaken in the tobacco industry.

> *"It is ... important to lay to rest ... the industry's assertion that nicotine is not addictive."*

It is equally important to lay to rest, once and for all, the industry's assertion that nicotine is not addictive. Up until very recently, the tobacco industry was able to claim that it did not believe that nicotine was addictive. The release of company documents, and the testimony of company scientists before this Subcommittee, has opened a window on what some senior tobacco officials knew about nicotine's physiological and addictive properties, as much as 30 years ago.

One important thing that every teenager in this country needs to know before deciding to smoke his or her first cigarette is how Addison Yeaman, a cigarette industry official, viewed the business of selling cigarettes in 1963: "We are, then, in the business of selling nicotine, an addictive drug ..."

Tobacco Companies Have Mounted Campaigns to Spread Smoking Worldwide

by Robert Weissman

About the author: *Robert Weissman is the editor of* Multinational Monitor, *a monthly magazine that reports on the practices of multinational corporations.*

Japanese multinational corporations may long ago have supplanted U.S. companies as the dominant economic power in Southeast Asia, but don't tell that to U.S. cigarette manufacturers. Their involvement in Southeast Asia is only in its early stages and it is growing rapidly.

Capitalizing on the worldwide fascination with U.S. culture and mythology, U.S. tobacco companies are aggressively hawking their cigarettes in the economically fast-growing region as the embodiment of U.S. lifestyle.

"Taste Kansas"

"Winston. Spirit of the U.S.A.," blared television commercials in the Philippines during telecasts of the U.S. professional basketball championship series in June 1993. Winston was the primary sponsor of the televised games, shown twice a day in June. The advertisements pictured healthy, vibrant, young Americans at play on the beach or the ballfield—smoking Winstons.

In Indonesia, billboards picturing rugged white men read "Lucky Strikes. An American Original." In imitation of the theme, signboards on display throughout the country for a local cigarette called "Kansas" urge potential consumers to "Taste America, Taste Kansas."

In Malaysia, the tobacco companies use the same themes. In an attempt to undermine and circumvent government anti-smoking initiatives—which include a ban on television advertisements for cigarettes—the tobacco companies sponsor

Robert Weissman, "Promoting the Tobacco Myth," *Multinational Monitor*, November 1993. Reprinted by permission.

televised events and use other businesses as fronts to promote their deadly product. Marlboro sponsors the "Marlboro World of Sports." Camel runs a clothing line. The British company Rothmans promotes its Peter Stuyvesant brand with billboards that picture images of the Statue of Liberty, American football players and cheerleaders and use a slogan connecting the brand name Stuyvesant to the magic word "America." Salem runs a music store, Salem Power Station, and a travel company, Salem World, which jointly took out full page advertisements in Malaysian newspapers in the summer of 1993 to promote a contest which had a trip to London to see a concert by the rock group U2 as its grand prize. The Salem brand name was prominently displayed in the advertisement, linked with the image of the band.

> *"[In Malaysia] Marlboro sponsors the 'Marlboro World of Sports.' Camel runs a clothing line. . . . Salem runs a music store."*

The effect of these advertising strategies, says Karen Lewis, manager of tobacco policy resources at the Washington, D.C.–based Advocacy Institute's Smoking Control Advocacy Resource Center, "is an increase in tobacco use and enormous increases in cancer mortality." The use of images that evoke "America" is particularly insidious, she contends, since it preys on poor people's longing for the political freedom and economic advancement popularly associated with the United States. "People want to be as American as they can be, if they associate it with being able to buy shoes."

The U.S. tobacco companies defend these advertising practices. While many of their advertising strategies might seem objectionable in the United States and some—notably television advertisements—would be illegal, "it is patently unfair to compare marketing and advertising practices of a given foreign country with the United States," says Brenda Follmer, director of public relations at R.J. Reynolds Tobacco International, the maker of both Winston and Salem brands. "It is the sovereign right of each government to establish its own laws and regulations. The reverse of this would be a foreign country dictating to the United States how it should regulate various industries. The respective governments establish their own laws and regulations, and companies must comply with those laws."

Moreover, argues Follmer, "it is a well-documented fact that all of these markets historically have had high rates of smoking."

Targeting Young People

But while tobacco use has long been widespread in Southeast Asia, says Lewis, "smoking in most traditional societies has been confined to adult men." In an effort to expand the market, the U.S. companies target women and young people, the groups which have historically had low smoking rates. "The focus on sports and rock concerts is obviously geared to young people," she says, and images of "American, thin, economically liberated women" are designed to entice women to take up the habit.

The tobacco companies deny targeting young people, with Follmer claiming that Reynolds "follows an internal policy of marketing our products exclusively to adult smokers, even in those markets where there is no minimum age requirement for purchasing or consuming cigarettes."

The slick advertisements based on sports, rock music and other elements of U.S. culture are only one component of the comprehensive marketing strategy pursued by the U.S. tobacco companies. Other elements, according to Lewis, range from shop-level strategies to industry-wide plans. Tobacco companies will offer to redecorate the entire exterior of a store or restaurant in exchange for the prominent display of the company's product and logo, and they may also provide interior point-of-sale displays. And they will strike similar deals with national tobacco companies, entering into joint ventures in which the U.S. company upgrades the national company's plants in exchange for a share of the company.

Even if they do not enter into joint ventures with foreign tobacco companies, national tobacco monopolies and private local companies respond to market pressures and begin to act more like the multinationals, imitating the U.S. corporations' Madison Avenue techniques and aggressive promotional tactics. Taken as a whole, the U.S. tobacco company strategy works to completely transform the national tobacco industries, even in countries where U.S. companies do not command major shares of the national market.

> *"There is little question that the U.S. tobacco companies' strategies pay dividends."*

There is little question that the U.S. tobacco companies' strategies pay dividends, as the results of the sudden introduction of U.S. cigarettes and tobacco company promotional techniques in the Korean market in 1988 make clear. In the year after the U.S. government forced Korea to lift import restrictions, the smoking rate among male teenagers rose by more than 50 percent, and among female teens by more than 300 percent, according to a U.S. General Accounting Office study.

Despite the eventual public health disaster the U.S. tobacco companies have virtually ensured for Southeast Asian countries in the decades to come, a much more frightening prospect looms on the horizon. These same companies are now working to knock down the trade barriers by which China limits foreign cigarette imports. Replication in that vast market of the tobacco companies' "success" in Southeast Asian countries would be a public health nightmare with few historical parallels.

Tobacco Companies Do Not Control the Nicotine Levels in Cigarettes

by William I. Campbell

About the author: *William I. Campbell is the president and chief executive officer of Philip Morris U.S.A., one of the largest cigarette manufacturers in the world.*

I would like to take this opportunity to set the record straight on charges that have recently been made against the industry and Philip Morris. First, Philip Morris does not add nicotine to our cigarettes. Second, Philip Morris does not "manipulate" or independently "control" the level of nicotine in our products. Third, Philip Morris has not used patented processes to increase or maintain nicotine levels. Fourth, cigarette smoking is not addictive. Fifth, Philip Morris has not hidden research which says that it is. And, finally, consumers are not misled by the published nicotine deliveries as measured by the FTC [Federal Trade Commission] method. . . .

The claim that cigarette smoking is addictive has been made for many years. The fact that tar and nicotine levels vary among our many products has been publicized for over 20 years. The process by which cigarettes are manufactured . . . has been publicly known for over 50 years. And the call for the FDA [Food and Drug Administration] to assert, or be given jurisdiction over cigarettes has been made and rejected by the FDA and the courts on several occasions in the past. . . .

Nicotine Is Not Added

The claim that Philip Morris secretly adds nicotine during the manufacturing process to "keep smokers addicted" is a false and irresponsible charge. The processes used to manufacture cigarettes have been publicly disclosed for years in patents and the published literature. And the results of that processing—

From William I. Campbell's statement before the House Committee on Energy and Commerce, Subcommittee on Health and the Environment, April 14, 1994.

cigarettes with varying levels of tar and nicotine reflecting varying customer preferences—have been closely monitored and reported by the FTC, and the manufacturers themselves in every advertisement, for 25 years.

Contrary to the claim that we are committed to maintaining, or even increasing, nicotine delivery in our products, the fact is that tar *and nicotine* levels have decreased dramatically over the past 40 years. Today, the market is populated with a number of "ultra low" brands which deliver less than 5% of the tar *and nicotine* of popular brands 20 years ago.

> *"Cigarette smoking is not addictive."*

Philip Morris and other manufacturers have reduced delivery in a number of ways. The most important is the use of increasingly efficient filters which substantially *reduce* many smoke components, including both tar *and nicotine*. Filtration reduces nicotine delivery 35% to 45% in today's brands, as compared to a "standard" cigarette made simply of tobacco and paper.

Through a process called ventilation, nicotine levels are reduced by 10% to 50%. Through the use of expanded tobacco—a process developed by Philip Morris, in which tobacco is "puffed" much like puffed rice cereal—tar and nicotine levels are reduced still further.

Reconstituted Tobacco

There has been a fair amount of recent discussion of the reconstituted tobacco process. Again, that process has been thoroughly described for years in the published literature. In that process, stems and small leaf parts are re-formed into a paper-like sheet. The reconstituted leaf process does *not* increase nicotine levels in tobacco or cigarettes. *To the contrary, 20% to 25% of the nicotine in the tobacco used to make reconstituted leaf is lost and not replaced.*

These processes, when combined in the cigarettes Philip Morris sells today, *reduce* nicotine delivery levels by more than 50% in the case of Marlboro, to 96% in the case of Merit Ultima, as compared to a "standard" cigarette made of nothing but tobacco and paper.

Ignoring these reductions, some critics have focused on minute amounts of nicotine that are found in tobacco extracts and denatured alcohol—which *together* have no measurable effect on nicotine delivery of our cigarettes.

Philip Morris uses denatured alcohol to spray flavors on the tobacco. The alcohol is denatured—that is, it is made to taste bitter so that no one will drink it —*under a formula required by the BATF* [Bureau of Alcohol, Tobacco and Firearms] *and found in the Federal Register.*

Again, the small amount of nicotine found in denatured alcohol and tobacco extracts cannot be measured in cigarette smoke.

The expenditure of millions of dollars to reduce tar and nicotine in these various ways undercuts any suggestion that Philip Morris is "intent" on adding nicotine to its cigarettes in an effort to "maintain" nicotine levels or to "addict" smokers.

We Don't Manipulate Nicotine

The cigarette industry markets and advertises products by tar category to satisfy a variety of consumer preferences. Within tar categories, we attempt to provide a competitive advantage by providing the best possible taste.

When creating a cigarette for a tar category, we select a particular tobacco blend and flavors to provide "uniqueness" for the product. The most significant parameters for determining tar delivery are the amount of expanded tobacco used, filtration efficiency, and ventilation.

So, how do we "manipulate" or independently "control" nicotine as our critics charge? *The answer is we don't.* We accept the nicotine levels that result from this process.

As representatives of the FDA learned when, at our invitation, they visited our manufacturing center in Richmond, nicotine levels in tobacco are measured at only two points in the manufacturing process—at the stemmery, where tobacco leaves are prepared for processing, and then *18 months later* after those leaves have been manufactured into finished cigarettes. Although Philip Morris maintains over 400 quality control checkpoints in the manufacturing process—for example, moisture levels, weight, etc.—*none* measures, reports or analyzes nicotine levels in tobacco.

Cigarette Smoking Is Not Addictive

Some . . . contend that nicotine is an addictive drug and that, therefore, smokers are drug addicts. I object to the premise and to the conclusion.

Many people like to smoke. Some people like the look and feel of the pack or the smell of tobacco. Some like to hold and fiddle with a cigarette. And, of course, there is the taste and aroma of the tobacco, and the sight of the smoke.

Cigarettes contain nicotine because it occurs naturally in tobacco. Nicotine contributes to the taste of cigarettes and the pleasure of smoking. The presence of nicotine, however, does not make cigarettes a drug or smoking an addiction.

> *"Tar and nicotine levels have decreased dramatically over the past 40 years."*

People can and do quit smoking. According to the 1988 Surgeon General's Report, there are over 40 million former smokers in the United States, and 90% of smokers quit on their own, without any outside help.

Further, smoking is not intoxicating. No one gets drunk from cigarettes, and no one has said that smokers cannot function normally. Smoking does not impair judgment. No one is likely to be arrested for driving under the influence of cigarettes.

In short, our customers enjoy smoking for many reasons. Smokers are not drug addicts.

Tobacco Ads Do Not Cause Teenagers to Smoke

by Jonathan Adler

About the author: *Jonathan Adler is a policy analyst at the Washington, D.C.–based Competitive Enterprise Institute, a public interest group dedicated to the principles of free enterprise and limited government.*

Responding to complaints filed by anti-smoking activists, the staff of the Federal Trade Commission [FTC] in 1993 called for banning cigarette advertisements featuring "Old Joe" Camel. . . .

The opposition to the Joe Camel advertising campaign is based upon allegations that R.J. Reynolds uses the character to induce minors to smoke. This, in turn, is labeled an "unfair" business practice because it is illegal for minors to purchase cigarettes. On these grounds, the Coalition on Smoking OR Health, which is made up of members of the American Lung Association, American Heart Association and the American Cancer Society, petitioned the FTC in late 1991 to "take immediate action against RJR's cartoon camel." The coalition was quickly joined in its campaign by other anti-smoking activists, including then-Surgeon General Antonia Novello. [The FTC subsequently rejected the ban, citing insufficient evidence that the ads cause minors to smoke. Ed.]

Irrelevant Findings

The cornerstone of the charges against the Joe Camel ad campaign is a series of studies published in the *Journal of the American Medical Association* in December 1991. The first of these studies allegedly showed that children were able to connect pictures of the Camel character to tobacco products. This is an interesting but largely irrelevant finding. That children can connect "Old Joe" with cigarettes says nothing about whether those children approve or disapprove of "Old Joe's" tobacco habit.

The second study attempted to estimate the percentage of underage smokers that smoke Camels, and that this percentage has increased since the introduc-

Abridged from Jonathan Adler, "Camel Hunting with the FTC," *Washington Times*, September 3, 1993. Reprinted with permission.

tion of the Camel campaign. In its defense, RJR points to figures that show that Camel's share of the total cigarette market has been relatively flat for the past several years.

The third study is the real center of the anti-Camel campaign. It is also this study that is of the most questionable validity. While its authors claimed that "Our study provides further evidence that tobacco advertising promotes and maintains nicotine addiction among children and adolescents," it actually did no such thing. As correspondence between the authors indicates, the data had been tailored by the authors to fit their predetermined conclusions.

The lead author of the study, Dr. Joseph R. DiFranza, was convinced that the Joe Camel campaign had "maximum appeal to boys about 11 years old," and that the campaign could be limited by producing "a couple of smoking guns to bring to the national media." This was the opinion he expressed in correspondence with colleagues. However, after conducting initial surveys, Dr. DiFranza found that his thesis was wrong and that the ads "appeal more to people in their 20s than in their early teens." This is what RJR had maintained all along. Dr. DiFranza wrote to his colleagues, "we have just disproved our theory that the ads appeal more to kids than to adults."

Skewing the Results

Still determined to tar the Camel campaign, the surveys were redone. This time, however, the age groups were manipulated so as to "demonstrate" that the ads had greater appeal to kids than adults. This was done by reducing the number of survey respondents in the 18–24 age range and adding much older respondents—one as old as 87—that would be less likely to find the ads appealing. The new study came to the "correct" conclusions, at the expense of scientific accuracy. It was this study that was published. Without it, the anti-smoking activists would have no case against Camel.

"The Joe Camel campaign has been subjected to criticism and allegations that would not be taken seriously against other, less-suspect, products."

Because cigarette smoking is a "politically incorrect" habit, the Joe Camel campaign has been subjected to criticism and allegations that would not be taken seriously against other, less-suspect, products. What is at stake is not whether a single company can freely advertise a legal product, but whether orchestrated campaigns against particular products will be rewarded with government bans. If this campaign is successful, it will set a dangerous precedent that could threaten consumer access to information and messages regarding a wide-range of "unpopular" products.

A vibrant marketplace relies upon the constant display and exchange of information. Advertising is the primary means for this exchange. It is how individuals and companies convey information about the range of products available to consumers. When advertising is limited, it not only has the potential to limit corporate profits, it also restricts the range of information that is available to the consumer.

Many find cigarette advertising distasteful because of their aversion to smoking. As a former smoker, I find this completely understandable. Nonetheless, it is misguided. Cigarette manufacturers and consumers should be afforded the same freedoms in the marketplace as is everyone else. So long as manufacturers refrain from fraud, their ability to communicate in this manner should not be proscribed.

Individuals Are Responsible for the Decision to Smoke

by Mona Charen

About the author: *Mona Charen is a conservative syndicated columnist whose articles appear in many national newspapers and magazines.*

I am no admirer of cigarette companies. They produce a product that is poisonous, and they peddle it in such a way as to make it glamorous. For years, they cheerfully accepted government subsidies. They are neither exemplary businessmen nor good capitalists.

A Farce

Still, the spectacle of histrionic Democratic congressmen haranguing the executives of the seven largest cigarette companies during 1994's hearings before the House Subcommittee on Health and the Environment was a farce.

Reps. Ron Wyden (D-Ore.), Henry Waxman (D-Calif.) and John Bryant (D-Texas), among others, taunted, interrupted and derided the tobacco makers, asking repeatedly whether cigarettes cause cancer, emphysema and heart disease. The executives responded that they couldn't say for sure.

In a sense, they have a point. No one can say for sure why a particular person comes down with lung cancer and another doesn't. Some people smoke two packs a day for 50 years and die of old age. But there are limitations to that kind of sophistry on the part of cigarette makers. What science has demonstrated conclusively is that there is a strong correlation between smoking and disease, making it safe to say that smoking is a risky behavior.

What exactly did the congressmen expect the tobacco executives to say? Everyone who has not been on Mars for the past 25 years knows that smoking increases the risk of contracting cancer and other diseases. The defensive stance of the tobacco industry is to hug agnosticism as close as they can this side of

Mona Charen, "Congressmen Know They Can't Ban Cigarettes," *Conservative Chronicle*, May 4, 1994. Reprinted by permission of Mona Charen and Creators Syndicate.

absurdity. Tobacco companies look silly trying to deny the danger of cigarettes, but theirs is not the only product on the market that can cause harm. Alcohol, when used to excess, can too. So can eggs, bacon and hollandaise sauce.

But millions of people, knowing the risks, choose to smoke anyway. The congressmen know that. They further know that they dare not ban cigarettes for fear of igniting either a revolution or a crime wave equal to or greater than that which accompanied Prohibition. (Imagine "smoke-easies.") Crime would probably be much worse now, considering the greater lawlessness of our society today.

Imaginary Crimes

Members of Congress have no intention of banning the sale of cigarettes. Nor do they endorse something useful, like the humorous British commercials urging smokers to empty their ashtrays into a large jar, fill it with water, and take a big sniff! Nor do they intend to mandate that smokers bear the brunt of their own higher insurance premiums. No, the self-righteous Democrats of the health subcommittee will do nothing to offend those of their constituents who smoke. The beauty of the hearing is that it permitted Reps. Waxman, Wyden et al. to invent villains—evil tobacco executives—and excoriate them for imaginary crimes.

Imaginary? Yes. The most telling moment of the hearings came when one of the congressmen asked the executives if cigarettes are addicting. "No," replied each of them in turn. This exchange made the evening news—presented in the light the politicians wanted. The executives were portrayed as outrageously disingenuous. Addiction "experts" were quoted contradicting the tobacco companies.

But we make entirely too much of the concept of addiction. Addiction is a physical process involving tolerance and certain symptoms upon withdrawal of the substance. All habits are hard to break. Addiction makes them harder to break. But it does not—as so many seem to assume—make habits impossible to break.

> *"Millions of people, knowing the risks, choose to smoke anyway."*

Even heroin addicts are known voluntarily to go through withdrawal when the price of their drug rises so that they can continue to get high on less.

"Millions of people want to quit smoking but can't," said one addiction expert on a morning show.

Well, that is a philosophical not a medical question. I quit smoking, after five years of a pack a day. It wasn't easy. Neither is losing weight. But it is eminently possible. Free will lives.

It makes better theater to pretend that evil tobacco companies are spiking their product with nicotine to keep people helplessly lighting up. The more mundane truth is that people are well-informed about the dangers of smoking and fully capable of stopping but smoke anyway.

Chapter 3

How Can Smoking Be Reduced?

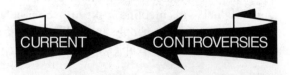
CURRENT CONTROVERSIES

Quitting Smoking: An Overview

by Carl Sherman

About the author: *Carl Sherman writes on health, medicine, and psychology for national magazines and medical newspapers.*

It may not be a "sin" anymore, but few would dispute that smoking is the devil to give up. Of the 46 million Americans who smoke—26 percent of the adult population—an estimated 80 percent would like to stop and one-third try each year. Two to 3 percent of them succeed. "There's an extraordinarily high rate of relapse among people who want to quit," says Michael Fiore, M.D., M.P.H., director of the Center for Tobacco Research and Intervention at the University of Wisconsin.

The tenacity of its grip can be matched by few other behaviors, most of which, like snorting cocaine and shooting up heroin, are illegal. Since 1988, nicotine dependence and withdrawal have been recognized as disorders by the American Psychiatric Association, legitimizing the experience of the millions who have tried, successfully and otherwise, to put smoking behind them while kibitzers told them to use more willpower.

Not Just a Habit

It's not just a habit, the medical and scientific communities now fully agree, but an addiction, comparable in strength to hard drugs and alcohol.

In fact, the odds of "graduating" from experimentation to true dependence are far worse for cigarettes than for illicit drugs, which testifies to tobacco's one-two punch of addictiveness and availability: Crack and heroin aren't sold in vending machines and hawked from billboards. Alcohol is as legal and available as cigarettes are, and as big a business, but apparently easier to take or leave alone. The majority of people who drink are not dependent on alcohol, while as many as 90 percent of smokers are addicted.

If nothing else, the persistence of smoking in the face of a devastating rogue's gallery of bodily damage, little of which has been kept secret, attests to the fact that this is no rational life-style decision. "Take all the deaths in America caused by alcohol, illicit drugs, fires, car accidents, homicide, and suicide. Throw in AIDS. It's still only half the deaths every year from cigarettes," says Fiore.

The news, however, isn't all bad. For the last 20 years, the proportion of Americans who smoke has dropped continuously, for the first time in our history. In America today, there are nearly 45 million ex-smokers, about as many as are still puffing away.

These quitters, perhaps surprisingly, are for the most part the same folk who tried and failed before. The average person who successfully gives up smoking does so after five or six futile attempts, says Fiore. "It appears that many smokers need to go through a process of quitting and relapsing a number of times before he or she can learn enough skills or maintain enough control to overcome this addiction."

The Effects of Smoking

Never underestimate the power of your enemy. Although nicotine may not give the taste of Nirvana that more notorious drugs do, its effects on the nervous system are profound and hard to resist. It increases levels of acetylcholine and norepinephrine, brain chemicals that regulate mood, attention, and memory. It also appears to stimulate the release of dopamine in the reward center of the brain, as opiates, cocaine, and alcohol do.

Addiction research has clearly established that drugs with a rapid onset—that hit the brain quickly—have the most potent psychological impact and are the most addictive. "With cigarettes, the smoker gets virtually immediate onset," says Jack Henningfield, Ph.D., chief of clinical pharmacology research for the National Institute on Drug Abuse. "The cigarette is the crack-cocaine of nicotine delivery."

Physiologically, smoking a drug, be it cocaine or nicotine, is the next best thing to injecting it. In fact, it's pretty much the same thing, says Henning-

> *"The average person who successfully gives up smoking does so after five or six futile attempts."*

field. "Whether you inhale a drug in 15 seconds, which is pretty slow for an average smoker, or inject it in 15 seconds, the effects are identical in key respects," he says. The blood extracts nicotine from inhaled air just as efficiently as oxygen, and delivers it, within seconds, to the brain.

The cigarette also gives the smoker "something remarkable: the ability to get precise, fingertip dose control," says Henningfield. Achieving just the right blood level is a key to virtually all drug-induced gratification, and the seasoned smoker does this adeptly, by adjusting how rapidly and deeply he or she puffs. "If you get the dose just right after going without cigarettes for an hour or two, there's nothing like it," he says.

Pain Relief

The impetus to smoke is indeed, as the tobacco companies put it, for pleasure. "But there's no evidence that smoke in the mouth provides much pleasure," says Henningfield. "We do know that nicotine in the brain does."

For many, nicotine not only gives pleasure, it eases pain. Evidence has mounted that a substantial number of smokers use cigarettes to regulate emotional states, particularly to reduce negative affect like anxiety, sadness, or boredom.

"People expect that having a cigarette will reduce bad feelings," says Thomas Brandon, Ph.D., assistant professor of psychology at the State University of New York at Binghamton. His research found this, in fact, to be one of the principal motivations for daily smokers.

Negative affect runs the gamut from the transitory down times we all have several times a day, to clinical depression. Smokers are about twice as likely to be depressed as nonsmokers, and people with a history of major depression are nearly 50 percent more likely than others to also have a history of smoking, according to Brandon.

> *"Depression appears to cut your chance of quitting by as much as one-half."*

Sadly, but not surprisingly, depression appears to cut your chance of quitting by as much as one-half, and the same apparently applies, to a lesser extent, to people who just have symptoms of depression.

According to Alexander Glassman, M.D., professor of psychiatry at the Columbia University College of Physicians and Surgeons, the act of quitting can trigger severe depression in some people. In one study, nine smokers in a group of 300 in a cessation program became so depressed—two were frankly suicidal—that the researchers advised them to give up the effort and try again later. All but one had a history of major depression.

"These weren't average smokers," Glassman points out. All were heavily dependent on nicotine, they smoked at least a pack and a half daily, had their first cigarette within a half hour of awakening, and had tried to quit, on average, five times before. It is possible, he suggests, that nicotine has an antidepressant effect on some.

More generally, suggests Brandon, the very effectiveness of cigarettes in improving affect is one thing that makes it so hard to quit. Not only does a dose of nicotine quell the symptoms of withdrawal (much more on this later), the neurotransmitters it releases in the brain are exactly those most likely to elevate mood.

For a person who often feels sad, anxious, or bored, smoking can easily become a dependable coping mechanism to be given up only with great difficulty. "Once people learn to use nicotine to regulate moods," says Brandon, "if you take it away without providing alternatives, they'll be much more vulnerable to negative affect states. To alleviate them, they'll be tempted to go back to what worked in the past."

Causes of Relapse

In fact, negative affect is what precipitates relapse among would-be quitters 70 percent of the time, according to Saul Shiffman, Ph.D., professor of psychology at the University of Pittsburgh. "We invited people to call a relapse-prevention hot line, to find out what moments of crises were like; what was striking was how often they were in the grip of negative emotions just before relapses, strong temptations, and close calls." A more precise study using palmtop computers to track the state of mind of participants is getting similar results, Shiffman says.

Most relapses occur soon after quitting, some 50 percent within the first two weeks, and the vast majority by six months. But everyone knows of people who had a slip a year, two, or five after quitting, and were soon back to full-time puffing. And for each of them, there are countless others who have had to fight the occasional urge, desire, or outright craving months, even years after the habit has been, for all intents and purposes, left behind.

Acute withdrawal is over within four to six weeks for virtually all smokers. But the addiction is by no means *all* over. Like those who have been addicted to other drugs, ex-smokers apparently remain susceptible to "cues," suggests Brandon: Just as seeing a pile of sugar can arouse craving in the former cocaine user, being at a party or a club, particularly around smokers, can rekindle the lure of nicotine intensely.

The same process may include "internal cues," says Brandon. "If you smoked in the past when under stress or depressed, the act of being depressed can serve as a cue to trigger the urge to smoke."

Psychological Impairment

Like users of other drugs, Henningfield points out, addicted smokers don't just consume the offending substance to feel good (or not bad), but to feel "right." "The cigarette smoker's daily function becomes dependent on continued nicotine dosing: Not just mood, but the ability to maintain attention and concentration deteriorates very quickly in nicotine withdrawal."

> *"For a person who often feels sad, anxious, or bored, smoking can easily become a dependable coping mechanism to be given up only with great difficulty."*

Henningfield's studies have shown that in an addicted smoker, attention, memory, and reasoning ability start to decline measurably just four hours after the last cigarette. This reflects a real physiological impairment: a change in the electrical activity of the brain. Nine days after quitting, when some withdrawal symptoms, at least, have begun to ease, there has been no recovery in brain function.

How long does the impairment persist? No long-term studies have been done, but cravings and difficulties in cognitive function have been documented for as long as nine years in some ex-smokers. "There are clinical reports of people who have said that they still aren't functioning right, and eventually make the 'rational decision' to go back to smoking," Henningfield says.

The conclusion is inescapable that smoking causes changes in the nervous system that endure long after the physical addiction is history, and in some smokers, may never normalize.

What Helps Smokers Quit

The wealth of recent knowledge about smoking clarifies why it's hard to quit. But can it make it easier? If nothing else, it should help people take it seriously enough to gear up for the effort. "People think of quitting as something short term, but they should expect to struggle for a couple of months," says Shiffman.

What works? About 90 percent of people who give up smoking do so on their own, says Fiore. But the odds for success can be improved: Programs that involve counseling typically get better rates, and nicotine replacement can be a potent ally in whatever method you use.

"The patch consistently doubled the success of quit attempts."

In a metaanalysis of 17 placebo-controlled trials involving more than 5,000 people, Fiore found that the patch consistently doubled the success of quit attempts, whether or not antismoking counseling was used. After six months, 22 percent of the people who used the patch remained off cigarettes, compared to 9 percent who had a placebo. Of those who had the patch and a relatively intense counseling or support program, 27 percent were smoke-free.

More than 4 million Americans have tried the patch, which replaces the nicotine on which the smoker has become dependent, to ease such withdrawal symptoms as irritability, insomnia, inability to concentrate, and physical cravings that drive many back to tobacco.

You're likely to profit from the patch if you have a real physical dependence on nicotine: that is, if you have your first cigarette within 30 minutes of waking up; smoke 20 or more a day; or experienced severe withdrawal symptoms during previous quit attempts.

Nicotine Maintenance

Standard directions call for using the patches in decreasing doses for two to three months. Some researchers, however, suggest that for certain smokers, the patch may be necessary for years, or indefinitely.

"It's already happening," says Henningfield. "Some doctors have come to the conclusion that some patients are best able to get on with their life with nicotine maintenance." One such physician is David Peter Sachs, M.D., director of the Palo Alto Center for Pulmonary Disease Prevention. "I realized that with some of my patients, no matter how slowly I tried to taper them off nicotine replacement, they couldn't do it," says Sachs. "They were literally using it for years. Before you start tapering the dose, you should be cigarette-free for at least 30 days."

His clinical experience leads him to believe that 10 to 20 percent of smokers are *so* dependent that they may always need to get nicotine from somewhere. One study of people using the gum found that two years later, 20 percent of those who had successfully remained cigarette-free were still chewing. The idea of indefinite, even lifetime, nicotine maintenance sounds offensive to some. "Clearly, the goal to aim for is to be nicotine-free," says Sachs. "But if that can't be reached, being tobacco-free still represents a substantial gain for the patient, and for society." And getting nicotine via a patch or gum source means a far lower dose than you'd get from a cigarette. Plus, you're getting just nicotine, and not the 42 carcinogens in tobacco smoke.

Although the once-a-day patch has largely supplanted the gum first used in nicotine replacement, Sachs thinks that for some, the most effective treatment could involve one or both. The patch may be easier to use, but the gum is the only product that allows you control over blood nicotine level. Some people know they'll do better if they stay in control. And would-be quitters who do fine on the patch until they run into a stressful business meeting may stifle that urge to bum a cigarette if they boost their nicotine level in advance with a piece of gum, Sachs says.

Coping Skills and Therapy

However, nicotine replacement "is not a magic bullet," says Fiore. "It will take the edge off the tobacco-withdrawal syndrome, but it won't automatically transform any smoker into a nonsmoker." Other requisite needs vary from person to person. A standard approach teaches behavioral "coping skills," simple things like eating, chewing gum, or knitting to keep mouth or hands occupied, or leaving tempting situations. Ways people cope cognitively are as important as what they do, says Shiffman.

He advises would-be quitters at times of temptation to remind themselves just why they're quitting: "My children will be so proud of me," or "I want to live to see my grandchildren," for example. Think of a relaxing scene. Imagine how you'll feel tomorrow if you pass this crisis without smoking. Or simply tell yourself, "NO" or "Smoking is not an option."

> *"Ten to 20 percent of smokers are* so *dependent that they may always need to get nicotine from somewhere."*

Coping skills, however, are conspicuously unsuccessful for people who are high in negative affect. Supportive counseling works better. Depression or anxiety may interfere with the ability to use cognitive skills.

One exercise that Brandon teaches patients asks them to inventory—and treat themselves to—things that make them feel good, a substitute for the mood-elevating effect of a cigarette. These might include exercising, being with friends, going to concerts, reading, or taking a nap. "Positive life-style changes that improve mood level" are particularly useful if you use cigarettes to deal with negative emotional states, he says.

Depression treatment is particularly important for those trying to quit smoking. One study found that cognitive therapy significantly improved quit rates for people with a history of depression. Various antidepressants have been effective in small studies, and a large double-blind trial using the drug Zoloft is underway.

Fiore has found that having just one cigarette in the first two weeks of a cessation program predicted about 80 percent of relapses at six months. Even when the withdrawal symptoms are gone, a single lapse can rekindle the urge as much as ever.

In the critical first weeks without cigarettes, a key to relapse prevention is avoiding, or severely limiting, alcohol, which not only blunts inhibitions, but is often powerfully bound to smoking as a habit. Up to one-half of people who try to quit have their first lapse with alcohol on board.

Watch your coffee intake, too. It can trigger the urge to smoke. And nicotine stimulates a liver enzyme that breaks down caffeine, so when you quit, you'll get more bang for each cup, leading to irritability, anxiety, and insomnia—the withdrawal symptoms that undermine quit efforts.

Try to change your routine to break patterns that strengthen addiction: drive to work a different way; don't linger at the table after a meal. And don't try to quit when you're under stress: vacation time might be a good occasion.

And if you do have a lapse? Don't trivialize it, because then you're more likely to have another, says Shiffman. But, "if you make it a catastrophe, you'll reconfirm fears that you'll never be able to quit," a low self-esteem position that could become a self-fulfilling prophecy. "Think of it as a warning, a mistake you'll have to overcome."

Try to learn from the lapse: examine the situation that led up to it, and plan to deal with it better in the future. "And take it as a sign you need to double your efforts," Shiffman says. "Looking back at a lapse, many people find they'd already begun to slack off; early on, they were avoiding situations where they were tempted to smoke, but later got careless."

Don't be discouraged by ups and downs. "It's normal to have it easy for a while, then all of a sudden you're under stress and for 10 minutes you have an intense craving," says Shiffman. "Consider the gain in frequency and duration: the urge to smoke is now coming back for 10 minutes, every two weeks, rather than all the time."

If lapse turns into relapse and you end up smoking regularly, the best antidote to despair is getting ready to try again. "Smoking is a chronic disease, and quitting is a process. Relapse and remission are part of the process," says Fiore. "As long as you're continuing to make progress toward the ultimate goal of being smoke-free, you should feel good about your achievement."

Physicians Can Help Patients Quit Smoking

by Thomas P. Houston

About the author: *Thomas P. Houston is director of the American Medical Association's Department of Preventive Medicine and Environmental Health.*

I understand that educating my patients about tobacco is important, but how do I incorporate this into my practice in a cost-effective way?

Counseling is crucial. As many as 70% of smoking patients report that firm, supportive messages from physicians can be an important motivating factor. Minimal-contact doctor counseling strategies are effective, time-efficient and personally rewarding. The four "A's" for smoking-cessation intervention are:

- Ask about smoking at every opportunity.
- Advise all smokers to stop.
- Assist patients in that effort.
- Arrange follow-up.

With children, a fifth "A" can be listed—anticipatory guidance to help keep kids from ever starting to smoke.

But there's much that you and your staff can do to educate patients before they enter the examining room.

The Office Setting

Take a look at the office setting with the eyes of a patient. Begin with the outside of the building or its entrance: A bus bench, billboard or poster featuring a humorous, innovative health promotion message about smoking can alert the patient to your philosophy.

Next, make sure that messages in the reception and waiting areas are consistent with the pro-health counseling that will follow. If the office uses magazines such as *Redbook, Cosmopolitan, Time, Sports Illustrated, Ladies Home Journal, Newsweek* or *Family Circle*, then patients are seeing advertisements telling them that smoking is glamorous, exciting, macho and associated with youth, success and health.

Some physicians only subscribe to magazines that refuse tobacco advertising. An alternative is to innovatively adapt the offensive advertising. For example, using a felt-tip marker to change "Benson and Hedges and Saturdays and me" to "Benson and Hedges and emphysema and me" turns the tables on the tobacco industry. One can easily "graffitize" all the unhealthy promotions in this manner.

Posters in the reception area, halls, toilets and exam rooms can continue to reinforce the health message. Ranging from the more traditional "Have a heart—don't smoke" to parody advertisements whose models dangle cigarettes from a nostril ("I smoke for smell") or feature bright yellow teeth ("They'll really know you're smoking"), posters really grab attention.

During the Exam

In the exam room, obtain the patient's smoking status as routinely as weight or blood pressure, and mark charts with a sticker on the cover to denote this status. The sticker will remind you to discuss cessation with all patients.

Designate an office staff member to act as smoking-cessation coordinator. It could become that person's responsibility to mark the charts for smoking status, replenish patient-education materials, graffitize magazine tobacco advertising and order posters, as well as to make the initial telephone follow-up contact with patients who have agreed to quit. Important attributes for this job are training in cessation counseling, good rapport with patients, skill in responding to patient anxieties and problems, and a commitment to the issue.

Coping with relapse is the most difficult aspect of smoking cessation for physicians and patients. The first two weeks of cessation are key to achieving success; relapses during this period strongly predict a return to smoking. Contact with patients should be made on or near the "quit date," about a week afterward and at the one-month anniversary of stopping. During follow-up, reinforce successful coping strategies, remind patients about methods to continue cessation and offer support if a slip occurs.

Patients often think relapse is associated with the doom of smoking forever. While many smokers will relapse after only one cigarette, others can be taught to learn from the slip and to avoid the situation that triggered smoking. Some common pitfalls include drinking alcohol (especially visits to bars), lack of support from friends and family and perceptions that the effects of cessation will be too hard to overcome.

> *"Firm, supportive messages from physicians can be an important motivating factor."*

The ex-smoker's belief in self-efficacy—but not the false impression that cessation is easy—is the best predictor of success. For those who relapse, encouragement to try again is important, since most smokers cycle through several tries before achieving success.

Nicotine Replacement Therapy Helps Smokers Quit

by Debra A. Mayer

About the author: *Debra A. Mayer is a research associate in epidemiology at the American Council on Science and Health, an association of scientists and physicians concerned with public health.*

With much fanfare, the nicotine transdermal delivery system, more commonly known as the "nicotine patch," was introduced in 1992. Approval by the Food and Drug Administration (FDA) was accompanied by an unprecedented direct marketing campaign by the pharmaceutical industry. In the ads, smokers were urged to ask their physicians about "the patch." Many heeded this call, with growing numbers reaching for a patch instead of a pack. With both the drug companies and smokers hopeful, nicotine patch sales of more than $1 billion were predicted for 1992.

One year later, the patch no longer appeared to be a "magical cure" for smoking addiction. Marketing experts expected patch sales in 1993 to fall to $250 million from $650 million in 1992. With large inventories and rampant discounting, 1994 sales were expected to fall below $175 million. These numbers are more a reflection of the formidable and complex nature of tobacco addiction than the failure of one particular smoking cessation aid. Although not a panacea, the nicotine patch is the most effective pharmacologic agent currently available to combat cigarette addiction. We need perspective on the strengths and shortcomings of this nicotine replacement therapy to approach smoking cessation programs with realistic expectations.

Nicotine Dependence

Nicotine is the agent responsible for the physically addictive nature of cigarettes. Within approximately eight seconds of inhalation, brain absorption

From Debra A. Mayer, "Nicotine Therapy: A Useful Tool in the Battle Against Smoking." Reprinted with permission from *Priorities* (vol. 6, no. 1, 1994), a publication of the American Council on Science and Health, 1995 Broadway, 2nd Floor, New York, NY 10023-5860.

of the chemical occurs, accounting for the "rush" smokers describe on initial inhalation. Because of this rapid brain penetration, smokers are able to self-medicate nicotine delivery. Nicotine is processed by the body rather quickly, so smokers need to have cigarettes throughout the day.

Nicotine affects multiple systems in the body. Withdrawal from this addictive drug is characterized by cravings, anxiety, irritability, hunger, restlessness, decreased concentration, drowsiness and sleep disturbance. These symptoms are generally most severe during the first one to two weeks of abstaining from tobacco use. The severity is associated with the level of the smoker's nicotine intake.

Nicotine Replacement

Nicotine replacement therapies were developed to alleviate some of these acute withdrawal symptoms. In addition to relieving the physical discomfort of smoking cessation, nicotine replacement offers a distinct health advantage. Although cigarette smoking is known to cause cancer, nicotine is not carcinogenic in either animals or humans.

Researchers realized that tobacco need not be the only vehicle to deliver nicotine to the body. Rather, nicotine could be administered in a controlled manner with the ultimate goal of reducing total drug intake. Because nicotine is inactivated during digestion, oral intake of the drug is an ineffective delivery method. Scientists needed to find other means by which nicotine could be absorbed into the body.

> *"The nicotine patch is the most effective pharmacologic agent currently available to combat cigarette addiction."*

Nicorette (Marion Merrell Dow), the nicotine gum, was one of the first replacement therapies developed. Available in 2 and 4 mg doses, the gum effectively releases nicotine into the mucosal lining of the mouth. Nicorette has been shown to be more effective than a placebo as an aid in smoking cessation, when used in conjunction with a behavior modification program. However, the main problem with Nicorette is limited patient compliance with the cessation program. Clinicians find that nicotine is not delivered in a very controlled manner. For example, even if patients chew adequate amounts of gum, they may still underdose themselves by not using the gum properly. They may chew it too quickly, and thus swallow most of the nicotine.

The Patch

The next development was the nicotine patch, which was designed to decrease withdrawal symptoms while addressing some of the shortcomings found with nicotine gum. There are four patches available for use in the U.S.: Habitrol (Ciba-Giegy), Nicoderm (Marion Merrell Dow), Nicotrol 16 (Johnson & Johnson) and Prostep (Lederle Laboratories). Although there are minor technical differences among the four types currently available, all produce their therapeutic effect by the same mechanism: The patches release a controlled amount of nicotine through the skin, where the drug is absorbed into the blood.

Nicotine patches differ from nicotine gum in several ways. One advantage of the patches is that they are "user-friendly"—once applied in the morning, they require little attention. The patches also produce steady serum levels of nicotine, rather than reinforcing the addictive nicotine "rush" normally experienced by smokers. Rates of successful cessation at the end of nicotine patch treatment, as well as long-term success rates, vary widely. However, quit rates among active nicotine patch users are consistently better than those of the placebo patch users in follow-up studies. For example, a review published in the *Journal of the American Medical Association* stated that overall success rates at six months ranged from 22 percent to 42 percent among active patch users compared with two percent to 28 percent among the placebo patch users. The research also suggests that the nicotine patch has significant impact on some of the previously described acute withdrawal symptoms associated with quitting smoking.

> *"Quit rates among active nicotine patch users are consistently better than those of the placebo patch users."*

The side effects reported from patch use are relatively mild. Local swelling at the patch site is reported in approximately three to eight percent of patch users. Approximately seven to 22 percent of patch users may experience redness at the patch site. Contrary to recent media reports, the patch is safe for use in patients with stable cardiovascular disease. However, patients who smoke while wearing the patch raise their risk of possible adverse effects of nicotine, including cardiovascular events. Patients need to understand that the patch is a substitute for smoking, and must not be used while smoking.

Where's the Magic?

The patches do not provide an easy cure for cigarette addiction. Smoking is a complex behavior, and nicotine addiction is only one part of the problem. In fact, smoking has at least three major addictive components: *habit, pleasure* and *self-medication*.

Habit refers to the fact that the more an individual engages in a certain behavior, the more likely the person is to repeat that behavior in the future. The behavior, smoking, automatically becomes part of a daily routine, a "natural" part of the day, associated with such common activities as talking on the phone, drinking a cup of coffee or driving a car. When trying to quit, smokers must relearn their daily routines and address this behavioral component of addiction. The nicotine patch does not help the smoker combat the habitual component of his or her addiction.

Individuals may also smoke to experience *pleasure*. As stated earlier, nicotine produces the smoker's "high" associated with cigarettes. By varying the rate of smoking, how deeply the smoke is inhaled and the length of time the smoke is held in the lungs, smokers are able to regulate their nicotine intake to optimize the pleasurable effects of the drug. The current dose-delivery system of the patch does not replace the pleasure derived from smoking. To address this problem, some companies may seek FDA approval to double the nicotine dose of the patches. Nicotine inhalers and sprays are also currently under development. These would more closely simulate the drug delivery system of cigarettes. Perhaps these newly designed nicotine replacement therapies will address this component of cigarette addiction.

Finally, people may smoke to *self-medicate* or reduce the unpleasant symptoms associated with tobacco withdrawal. Nicotine replacement therapy is most effective at treating this aspect of smoking addiction.

The Crucial Role of Therapy

Studies indicate that nicotine replacement therapies are most effective when used in conjunction with additional support services. For example, in one study in which minimal support services were used with the patch, success rates (measured as total abstinence from cigarettes) for active patch treatment at one year were 17 percent. In comparison, when a research group combined patch use with an intensive behavior therapy program, success rates at one year were 35 percent for active patch users. Looking at the success rates in two different studies is not the most accurate way to compare the use of patches with or without adjuvant therapy. But until better studies are done, this research does support the usefulness of incorporating nicotine patches into a more comprehensive smoking cessation plan.

Quit for Life—It's Worth the Investment!

The development of effective aids for smoking cessation is a critical public health concern. Smokers need to understand that quitting provides major and immediate health benefits. Each year, approximately 1.3 million smokers quit successfully. If nicotine replacement therapy does not prove to be the smoker's weapon of choice, there are many other types of smoking cessation programs. Physicians need to encourage their patients to find the method that works best for them. A short period of discomfort will be rewarded with many years of a more active, healthy life.

Smokers Must Use Willpower to Quit Smoking

by Leonard Larsen

About the author: *Leonard Larsen is a columnist for the Scripps Howard News Service.*

If cigarette smokers—real pack-a-day-plus people who've smoked for many years—need a nicotine nasal spray to help them quit smoking, they probably aren't ready to quit and they won't quit.

The notion is as foolish as nicotine patches or nicotine gum to make smokers quit or magic charms or $25 sessions in crowded motel rooms while quack psychologists try to get your mind off smoking.

An ultimate foolishness is that the nicotine spray now comes recommended by non-smokers and never-been-smokers at the Food and Drug Administration who seem more intent on giving cigarette smokers crutches for their "addiction" than enough backbone to just quit.

Demonizing the Industry

The new nicotine nasal spray—to be available only by prescription—fits nicely with the demonization of tobacco company officials by the FDA and a few members of Congress. Not satisfied with emphasizing the plain truth that cigarettes are proved to be cancer-causing and a dangerous long-term habit that should be ended and never started, the demonologists have spent lavishly in time and money to prove other things.

Great evil conspiracies have been at work to turn little children into cigarette addicts, the public servants have said every time a TV camera was in their vicinity. The proof, said the non-smoking experts, was in reports that the conspirators tinkered with nicotine content in cigarettes and baited helpless tots with irresistible advertising of a smoking camel.

Louder now than the message that Americans should quit smoking because it might kill them is the demonologists' message that someone else is to blame

Leonard Larsen, "Blowing Away the Smoking Demons," *Washington Times*, March 31, 1996. Reprinted by permission of Scripps Howard News Service, a subsidiary of United Media.

for your smoking habit. The tobacco industry conspirators, as the propaganda line now runs, have hooked millions of Americans on cigarettes, just as they always intended, and the addicted victims are helpless to cure themselves.

So the wrongheaded officials of the FDA and grandstanders in Congress—aided by pack media specialists—end up sounding alarms and finger-pointing at a tobacco conspiracy instead of actually helping cigarette smokers quit.

Worse, they spread the nonsense that all smokers are "addicts," that they can't quit, that addicted smokers need crutches like arm patches or gum or now a nicotine nasal spray that's supposed to satisfy the cravings of cigarette addicts until they can get all the way unhooked.

That's no way to get people to quit smoking. It's giving smokers an excuse to keep on smoking. And, as a onetime smoker who spent about 42 years buying and smoking—and enjoying—cigarettes before I quit, I'll stack that experience alongside whatever arguments the expert non-smokers bring to the subject.

No Device Needed

To quit smoking, I found, doesn't require any device, and the study results on tests of the nasal spray released by the FDA would seem to support that conclusion. The studies, it was said, found that only 25 percent of smokers given the nasal spray quit smoking for at least a year, about the same results as smokers who used nicotine patches or chewed nicotine gum.

To quit smoking, I found, you have to make up your mind that you want to quit and that you're going to quit, not that you'll try to quit or quit the first of next month or think about quitting a little longer.

"If cigarette smokers ... need a nicotine nasal spray to help them quit smoking, they probably aren't ready to quit."

I came to an understanding that smoking cigarettes was at least partly a ceremony for me, a ceremony I enjoyed when relaxing over a cup of coffee or something stronger, even enjoyed at work writing. I liked the smell of it, the sight of exhaled smoke and smoke curling off a cigarette. I liked smoking and conversation with friends.

Then I began thinking—I knew—that smoking was a health hazard and increasingly bothersome to other people. I decided to give up the habit, the ceremony I enjoyed. I quit; no nasal sprays or arm patches and no humbuggery from the FDA. Just like millions of other people, I just quit.

It may be that the experts at the FDA intend to pursue their tobacco conspiracy until the culprits are all locked up in prison. Fine. But it won't help any of the smokers who've been convinced by the FDA that they're addicts and need crutches.

Women's Organizations Can Help Women Quit Smoking

by Sharon Lerner

About the author: *Sharon Lerner is a New York City–based freelance writer and editor. She frequently writes on health care issues.*

Seventy-five years ago, a woman ran for president of the United States on an antismoking platform. Lucy Page Gaston, who ran against known smoker Warren G. Harding, thought that smoking led to drinking, a life of crime, and a condition she called "cigarette face." She objected particularly to smoking by minors and women and, with the support of a substantial turn-of-the-century antismoking movement, she helped restrict smoking in more than 20 states by the mid-1920s. At the time, women accounted for an estimated 5 percent of all tobacco consumers.

We've come a long way since then, of course. Women now make up nearly half of all smokers in the U.S. (48 percent), and researchers predict we will soon be the majority. The number of females who begin smoking during high school and college has risen steadily, while the number of males has declined. And recent studies on smoking trends show that women as a group—in particular women living in poverty and those with less education—are doing worse with smoking than the overall population.

What is perhaps most upsetting about these landmarks is that we reach them in the face of overwhelming evidence that smoking does cause disease—things far worse than "cigarette face." While men have thus far dominated the habit during a period of ignorance about health effects, women are poised to become the majority of smokers at a time when it's absolutely clear that smoking is harmful.

Ignoring the Medical Evidence

At least part of the problem is that it's still not widely understood just how harmful it is to smoke. Many people still lump it in with risks like pesticides on fruit or sunbathing. The truth is that smoking kills more women than alcohol, illicit drugs, car accidents, suicide, and homicide—*combined*. It's by far the number one cause of premature death in women, causing approximately 20 percent of *all deaths*, killing roughly one in seven—or 141,832—women annually. Lung cancer, which has increased over 400 percent in women in the past 30 years, is now the biggest cancer killer of women—bigger even than breast cancer. And together, conditions such as emphysema, heart disease, stroke, and various other cancers are responsible for more smoking-related deaths than lung cancer.

There is now also overwhelming evidence that women are uniquely vulnerable to certain smoking-related health problems. Women smokers are

> *"Women are uniquely vulnerable to certain smoking-related health problems."*

more susceptible to reproductive tract infections and cervical cancer, and those who use oral contraceptives have an especially high risk of stroke and heart disease. Smoking also wreaks havoc on women's hormonal systems—decreasing fertility, increasing the chances of premature menopause and osteoporosis, and disrupting pregnancy. Women smokers have more preterm stillbirths, and their children are more likely to suffer and die from a variety of birth defects.

If the full extent of the above litany is not common knowledge, most of us have gotten the basic message: smoking is bad for you. Nevertheless, the medical news about smoking has had far less impact on women's smoking than on men's. Middle-class white men have stopped smoking in greater numbers than any other group, while women's smoking has gone down only slightly overall.

Starting Young

Why have female smokers been so unresponsive to the grim health news? A large part of the answer, according to Jean Forster, a researcher at the University of Minnesota School of Public Health, lies in the fact that most smokers—over 90 percent—take up the habit before age 20. African American girls constitute the one exception to this rule. The smoking rate among black teenagers has dropped in the past 10 to 15 years, but the rate significantly increases for black women later in life. Researchers have yet to reach a consensus as to why African American women often start smoking at a later age.

The average teen smoker begins at age 13. "At that point," says Forster, who has conducted focus groups with teenage smokers, "the public health message means nothing to kids. They're simply too young for it." And the earlier people start, the more likely they are to smoke heavily and the harder it will be for them to quit. But according to Forster, most teenagers are not worried about that. They are confident they will quit before they develop health problems, even before they become addicted. And, for teenage girls especially, concerns such as social acceptance, attractiveness, and body image often far outweigh thoughts of serious illness in the far-off future.

Advertising and Promotion

Cigarette marketers' ability to appeal to these concerns has been critical to their success in replacing the two to three million smokers who either quit or die each year. With the industry now spending over $4 billion annually on advertising and promotion (after cars, cigarettes are the second most advertised consumer product in the U.S.—despite the fact that cigarette advertising is banned from broadcast media), marketing techniques have reached a new level of complexity. Lately, many brands have taken to offering products geared to women that can be bought with proofs of purchase from cigarette packs. These incentives are offered with a time limit, so that you have to buy 400 packs of Merits within six months, for example, to get the "Merit Award" of a suede barn jacket. For the outfit featured in Virginia Slims' V-wear ad, you have to buy about five and a half packs a day for six months, according to the calculations of Dr. Elizabeth Whelan, president of the American Council on Science and Health, who keeps close track of cigarette ads aimed at women.

While cigarette companies regularly devise new marketing gimmicks such as these, the main themes of their ads have remained the same since they began marketing to women and girls about 70 years ago. One longtime favorite, the association of smoking with independence, equality, and, yes, feminism, dates back to when women's smoking was socially unacceptable. Tobacco marketers capitalized on the allure of breaking that taboo, casting cigarettes as a symbol of women's liberation: one public relations agent even arranged for a contingent of women to march in the 1929 New York City Easter parade carrying "little torches of freedom." To this day, variations on the theme that smoking makes women tough, independent, and equal to men surface in ads—especially in Virginia Slims ads, from "You've come a long way, baby" to the recent "You can do it" slogan.

Cigarettes and Thinness

Another recurrent theme of cigarette marketing to women—identifying smoking with being thin—began with Lucky Strikes' 1920s "Reach for a Lucky instead of a sweet" ad, which featured a slim woman with a shadow of a double chin looming behind her. Female models in cigarette ads still conform to standard ideals of beauty, including thinness. And ads often emphasize the words "slim" and "thin," as in the Capri slogan "There is no slimmer way to smoke" and Misty's "slim and sassy." As a result, according to former Surgeon General C. Everett Koop, many young girls are left with the misconception that taking up smoking will actually make

> *"For teenage girls especially, concerns such as social acceptance, attractiveness, and body image often far outweigh thoughts of serious illness."*

them thin. "Most of the adolescent female smokers I have talked with tell me they smoke to prevent gaining weight," says Koop, who has traveled extensively throughout the country interviewing young smokers. "They believe that if women who stop smoking gain weight, smoking must be a preventive to weight gain as well."

> *"Many young girls are left with the misconception that taking up smoking will actually make them thin."*

But regardless of content, the presence of cigarette ads alone influences women by affecting the editorial policies of the publications that carry them. It's now widely known that magazines that accept cigarette ads are less likely to report on the health effects of smoking, and studies have shown that tobacco ad revenue has an even greater impact on health reporting in women's magazines than in other publications.

Tobacco funding also complicates antismoking efforts by women's professional and political groups. Unfortunately the practice is unlikely to change given the scarcity of funding for women's organizations and the good publicity it affords the tobacco companies. Betty Dooley, president of the Women's Research and Education Institute, says that without the support of the tobacco industry, the organization would be unable to continue its public policy fellowship program—the only one of its kind for women. Spokesman K. Richmond Temple insists that Philip Morris' motivation for funding women's groups comes from its female employees, who "support women's participation in all aspects of life."

Staying Smoking

While the image of smoking has much to do with its initial appeal, the *experience* of smoking is, of course, why people continue to smoke. Smoking is pleasurable. It can relax muscles, increase concentration, and relieve anxiety. Because women are more likely to live in poverty and juggle multiple roles, these physical effects hold particular appeal as ways to reduce stress and to exert control over their environment. Lorraine Greaves, vice president of the International Network of Women Against Tobacco and a sociologist who has analyzed the many ways smoking functions for women, notes that it can provide them with an escape when no others exist. "Women often smoke to claim and mark their personal space," says Greaves. "This allows them to separate or break from partners, children, and workmates whenever desired."

The special social significance of smoking to women may explain the gender differential in quitting success. According to the Centers for Disease Control's 1993 National Health Interview Survey, slightly more women than men want to quit completely (73 percent as opposed to 67 percent, respectively), while slightly fewer female smokers (46.7 percent as opposed to 51.9 percent) are successful in their attempts.

But the reality is that it's extraordinarily difficult for anyone to quit, mostly because tobacco is incredibly physically addictive (despite what some tobacco executives say). As Jack Henningfield, a scientist at the National Institute on Drug Abuse, sees it, although gender-related pressures may add to women's difficulties in quitting, the main problem is simply being exposed to nicotine. "All the advertising in the world wouldn't affect women if nicotine weren't addictive," says Henningfield. "Just having a normal, healthy, functioning brain means that you are prewired to be a nicotine addict."

Slaying the Giant

Many in the antismoking movement look to regulatory possibilities—such as further restricting advertising, tightening youth access, limiting public smoking, and classifying and regulating tobacco as a drug—as their best hopes. But with annual revenues of $48 billion at stake, the industry is a daunting opponent, and so far it has managed to preserve its profits by creatively circumventing restrictions. When tobacco ads were banned from radio and TV in 1971, for instance, the industry compensated by stepping up other ad efforts; the relative share of tobacco ad revenue in women's magazines soared after this point—it more than tripled from 1967 to 1986. And many see the current trend of expanding sales into the "developing" world as a direct result of increased restrictions in the "developed" world.

The 1994 Republican electoral landslide, made possible in part by $1 million in campaign contributions from tobacco companies, allowed the industry to yet again avoid serious regulation. In addition to the strong antiregulatory tenor of this current Congress, the November 1994 election brought a shift in leadership that bodes badly for tobacco regulation. Representative Henry Waxman (D.-Calif.), who oversaw the recent investigation of industry manipulation of nicotine levels, has been deposed—and the investigation halted. The person who now has control over almost all tobacco-related regulation is Representative Thomas Bliley, Jr. (R.-Va.), who (until redistricting in 1990) represented a congressional district in which Philip Morris is the largest employer. During the 1994 election, Bliley received more contributions from tobacco industry political action committees than any other member of the House.

> *"Gender-related pressures may add to women's difficulties in quitting."*

Although a few optimistic health advocates see potential for bipartisan support of tobacco control by casting it as a "pro-family" issue, most have a grimmer outlook, at least for the moment. But while the possibilities may be bleak in Washington, D.C., women are increasingly active and successful in fighting tobacco on other levels. Such organizations as the Berkeley, California-based Women and Girls Against Tobacco, the American Medical Women's Association, and NOW [National Organization for Women], as well as a growing network of international women's organizations, have recently begun major outreach projects to raise consciousness about the tobacco issue. And people all over the country are fighting the image war, covering cigarette ads with their own antismoking stickers and putting up counter-ads, such as a "Virginia Slime" campaign that recently ran in the New York City subway system. The point, of course, is to heighten women's personal and collective awareness that smoking has more to do with being exploited than with being liberated.

Increased Taxes on Cigarettes Would Reduce Smoking

by Teh-Wei Hu et al.

About the author: *Teh-Wei Hu is a professor of health economics in the School of Public Health at the University of California at Berkeley.*

Proposition 99, the California Tobacco Tax and Health Promotion Act of 1988, was enacted by voters in November 1988, and became law on January 1, 1989. The initiative amended the state constitution, increasing the tax on cigarettes and other tobacco products by 25 cents, from 10 cents to 35 cents per pack. It also specified how these revenues may be used.

Allocation of Funds

A health education account receives 20 percent of the revenues "for programs for the prevention and reduction of tobacco use, primarily among children, through school and community health education programs" [according to a 1990 report in the *Journal of the American Medical Association*]. Hospitals and physicians who provide services for patients who cannot afford to pay receive 45 percent of funds, 5 percent are for research, and 5 percent are for parks, recreation and environmental programs. The remaining 25 percent of the revenues are placed in an unallocated account, to support any of these programs and fire prevention activities.

The legislature has appropriated some $125 million a year from the health education account. Funds have been appropriated to the state Department of Education, which has given grants to school districts to create school-based programs designed to discourage children from smoking.

The state Department of Health Services supervises the use of the remaining education funds used for tobacco control. About $15 million a year has been used in an anti-smoking media campaign. Media include television, radio,

Excerpted from "The Impact of Proposition 99, a Major Antismoking Law, on Cigarette Consumption" by Teh-Weh Hu, Jushan Bai, Theodore E. Keeler, Paul G. Barnett, and Hai-Yen Sung, *Journal of Public Health Policy*, Spring 1994. Reprinted with permission.

newspapers and billboards. Some of the advertising has been targeted to communities of ethnic and racial minorities. Also funded have been programs of grants to local health departments, and a competitive grants program that funds projects proposed by community agencies. All these programs are concerted efforts to control tobacco use in California.

A Decline in Smoking

Several studies have reported the declining smoking prevalence after implementation of Proposition 99, based on either state cigarette sales data, the California Tobacco Survey, or the Behavioral Risk Factor Survey conducted by the Department of Health Services in collaboration with the Centers for Disease Control. An earlier study, based on the two years (1989 and 1990) after Proposition 99, concluded that the California tax reduced cigarette consumption by slightly less than 5 percent to 7 percent, but was not able to differentiate the short-term from the long-term effects of the tax increase. The California Tobacco Survey reported that the prevalence of cigarette smoking among adults in California was reduced from 26.7 percent in 1988, in the pre-Proposition period, to 22.2 percent in 1992. This reduction in smoking prevalence rates is a significant indication of the impact of California Proposition 99.

"Several studies have reported the declining smoking prevalence after implementation of Proposition 99."

This viewpoint reports the magnitude of the effect of Proposition 99 on cigarette sales between January 1989 and December 1991, both in terms of the immediate effect and the long-term effect, due to the tax increase and/or other anti-smoking initiatives provided by the legislation. At the same time, this viewpoint plans to provide policy analysis and implications so that policymakers on anti-smoking legislation in California, as well as other states in the country, may learn from this legislation. . . .

Taxation and Consumption

Cigarette sales data are obtained from the California State Board of Equalization, reported on the basis of monthly sales of cigarette tax stamps. In this viewpoint we assume that the sale of a tax stamp is equivalent to the consumption of a single pack of 20 cigarettes. To avoid the influence of the 1983 Federal cigarette excise tax increase we began our data series in January 1984 and ended it in December 1991. The series includes 36 months after the implementation of the Proposition 99 tax, a period sufficiently long to display the impact of the tax on cigarette consumption. It should be noted, however, that beginning January 1991 there was a Federal excise tax increase of 4 cents per pack. In estimating the short-term and long-term effects of Proposition 99, we have taken into account the Federal tax and also have compared the different effects of the state tax and the Federal tax. Consumption is expressed as packs per civilian adult. . . .

The analysis shows that since 1984 there has been a continuous decline in the per capita cigarette consumption, whether in absolute terms (-0.034 packs per capita per month) or in percentage terms (-0.3 percent). The results also indicate that there was a significant increase in cigarette sales (1.03 packs per capita or a 10 percent increase) in the month following the passage of Proposition 99 (December 1988).

The predicted effects of Proposition 99 over the three-year period (1989–1991), based on the estimated time-series model, are presented in Figure 1 (the dotted line indicates the predicted values had there been no Proposition 99). We found that the immediate effect was very large: per capita sales were reduced by 2 packs or a 25.7 percent decline in January 1989 from expected sales in the absence of Proposition 99. This drastic decline can partly be explained by the increase in sales in December 1988 by one pack or 10 percent per adult capita. [Since Proposition 99 was passed in November 1988, but did not go into effect until January 1989, retailers and consumers probably purchased additional cigarettes during November and December 1988 in anticipation of the January 1, 1989 tax increase.] This drastic immediate effect declined very quickly. By June 1989 (six months later), the sales had only declined by 0.94 packs or 10.9 percent, and by the end of 1989 and throughout 1991, per capita sales declined by 0.75 packs or 9.5 percent. Thus the estimated long-term effect of Proposition 99 was maintained at a 9.5 percent reduction rate after three years. When these monthly differences are multiplied by the number

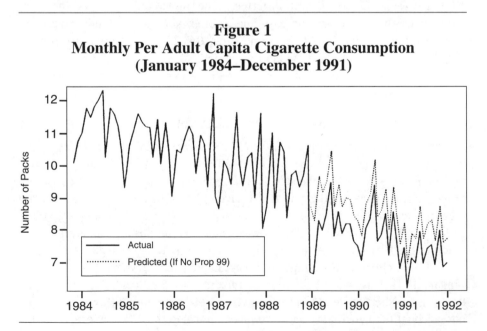

Figure 1
Monthly Per Adult Capita Cigarette Consumption
(January 1984–December 1991)

of the adult population in California during the three-year period, Proposition 99 reduced cigarette consumption by approximately 705 million packs between January 1989 and December 1991.

The 4-cent increase in the Federal tax on cigarettes during 1991 had a significant effect throughout the year, a 0.28 packs reduction in cigarettes sales. The relative magnitude of the effect of the Federal tax compared to the effect of the state tax, with respect to the amount of tax increase (4 cents versus 25 cents), suggests that Federal tax is stronger than state tax in terms of reducing cigarette consumption. The stronger effect of Federal tax than state tax could be due to the elimination of interstate cigarette smuggling, and also the potentially more visible announcement effect of the Federal tax increase at the national level. In spite of the effectiveness of the Federal tax imposed in 1991, the effectiveness and magnitude of the impact of Proposition 99 was not diminished or reduced. This study has compared the results before the Federal tax period (1984–1990) and the period including the Federal tax (1984–1991). . . . The estimated effect of Proposition 99 has maintained a 9 percent reduction rate after three years.

Taxes Reduce Cigarette Use

The findings from this study show that Proposition 99 was effective in reducing cigarette consumption. The Proposition had two effects, a temporary 16 percent decline in consumption, which quickly eroded, and an additional long-term effect, a 9 percent decline, which persisted throughout the remaining next three years. This pattern of decline can be best depicted by Figure 2, which provides a trend line before and after Proposition 99. The erosion of the temporary

Figure 2
Trend of Monthly Per Adult Capita Cigarette Sales—
With and Without Proposition 99

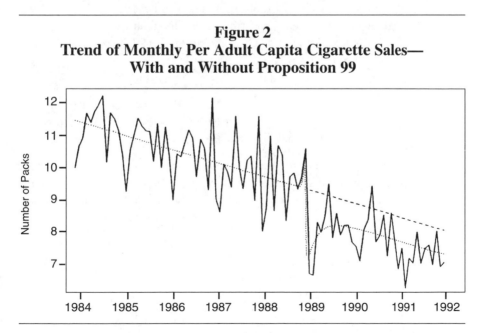

effect can be explained by the depletion of stocks of hoarded cigarettes, by the addictive nature of cigarette smoking behavior, and by the slight erosion of the tax by inflation. Thus the tax deterred the consumption more in the short-run than long-run. . . .

To sustain the effect of cigarette taxes, it would be appropriate to increase the cigarette tax periodically, or to assess them on an ad valorem basis [as a percent of value]. There have been complementary activities in smoking prevention funded by the revenue generated by Proposition 99. These activities, which began mid-1990, include an educational program and a media campaign for smoking prevention. In addition, most Californians now live in a jurisdiction where local ordinances regulate smoking in public places such as restaurants. It is difficult to separate the effect of taxation from the effect of the media and educational campaigns during the 36-month period. Thus this study provides an overall picture of the reduction of cigarette consumption since Proposition 99, and does not claim that the reduction is due solely to the 25-cent tax increase.

The findings from the 1991 Federal tax on cigarettes suggest that it has an additional effect on reduction of cigarette consumption and that its effect is quite strong. To achieve greater results in reducing cigarette consumption, the Federal government should take a more aggressive role to impose additional Federal tax on cigarettes. . . .

The use of cigarette tax revenue for medical care services has often been justified because of the external excess medical cost of smoking. Proposition 99 increased the total Federal and state excise taxes in California from 26 cents per pack in 1988 to 51 cents per pack beginning in 1989. The increased tax in California could almost cover the external excess medical cost of smoking, according to the estimates at the 1990 level from T.A. Hodgson ($0.47 per pack for male and $0.58 for female), and W.G. Manning et al. ($0.40 per pack). However, additional factors must be considered in estimating the economic burden of cigarette smoking such as lost productivity due to illness and disability, lost earnings from premature deaths, costs incurred due to passive smoking, accidents due to smoking-related fires, and so on. When these indirect costs are estimated, excess economic costs associated with smoking could reach anywhere from $1.00 per pack to as high as $5.23 per pack.

> *"Since 1984 there has been a continuous decline in the per capita cigarette consumption."*

Banning Tobacco Ads on Billboards Would Reduce Smoking

by Donald W. Garner

About the author: *Donald W. Garner is a professor at the Southern Illinois University School of Law in Carbondale.*

When, in 1990, the improbably named Rev Calvin Butts led his Abyssinian Baptist congregation in a widely reported campaign to whitewash tobacco and alcohol billboards that litter the streets of Harlem, he inspired a national movement. As activists in other cities emulated his tactics, state and local politicians were prompted to take a fresh look at the long-standing problem of intrusive tobacco advertising.

Bold Action

Although Kentucky and Texas responded by passing laws requiring that tobacco billboards be kept a certain distance from schools and churches, the city of Baltimore, Md, was the first to take bold and decisive action. In 1994, it completely banned "publicly visible" cigarette and alcoholic beverage advertisements except on "property adjacent to an interstate highway," in heavy industrial zones, and at Baltimore's Memorial Stadium. Now, only about 70 billboards, out of more than 1,000 in the city, can legally display these ads.

Baltimore is on the cutting edge of a growing movement by federal, state, and local governments to limit those forms of tobacco advertising that involuntarily assault the public with their message. For instance, on March 1, 1996, a new billboard ordinance in Cincinnati, Ohio, went into effect that will get rid of many outdoor tobacco signs in the city's neighborhoods by preventing their displays near schools, parks, and playgrounds. California now prohibits tobacco advertising on state buildings and in video games. Many cities now ban tobacco advertising in sports arenas and on public transit systems. A few small towns—

Preston, Minn, Millis, Mass, and neighboring communities—enacted prohibitions on indoor point-of-sale tobacco advertising, although they have subsequently encountered legal roadblocks.

The Food and Drug Administration and President Bill Clinton have climbed onto the bandwagon by proposing, among other things, to restrict all "advertising that reaches children," including billboard and point-of-sale advertising, to a "black and white, text-only format." The proposed regulations would also prohibit even these no-color, no-image billboards within 1,000 feet of schools and playgrounds.

A Cheap Way to Reduce Demand

The popularity of these measures is not hard to explain. Laws that eliminate or restrict tobacco billboard and outdoor sign advertising offer the particularly happy prospect of reducing juvenile demand for tobacco products without raising taxes, burdening police, creating another school program, or angering smokers. The only drawback is the prospect of having to defend such laws in court against the tobacco corporations and their allies, who may challenge them on the ground that they violate the First Amendment and are preempted by federal law.

However, Baltimore's foray onto new legal terrain has cleared a wide path for others to follow. Baltimore was sued by a billboard company, Penn Advertising, that sought to enjoin enforcement of the tobacco ordinance on First Amendment and federal preemption grounds. The city successfully repelled these challenges in federal district court and in the US Court of Appeals for the Fourth Circuit. Its alcohol billboard ordinance has also been upheld against a similar First Amendment challenge. Indeed, in both the tobacco and the alcohol billboard cases, Baltimore prevailed on a motion for summary judgment, ie, it won without the trouble and expense of going to trial.

> *"The Supreme Court knows the difference between the marketplace of products and the marketplace of ideas."*

The Fourth Circuit Court of Appeals' unanimous endorsement of the Baltimore ordinances now provides even the most cautious city council or state legislature with an influential precedent that can help guide their tobacco advertising restrictions between the Scylla of the First Amendment and the Charybdis of federal preemption.

The First Amendment Issue

Commercial speech, ie, advertising, was at one time accorded no First Amendment protection. However, in V*irginia State Board of Pharmacy v Virginia Citizens Council Inc*, the Supreme Court let commercial speech into the First Amendment stable, if not the manor. *Virginia Pharmacy* presented a perfect opening for the Supreme Court to grant at least some protection to commercial advertising. The state of Virginia had blatantly attempted to protect drugstores from price competition by prohibiting pharmaceutical price advertising. The Supreme Court knocked down this special-interest scheme as a burden on the right of Virginia's poor and infirm to know where to find the lowest price for their medication. However, Justice Harry Blackmun's majority opinion sensibly refused to equate advertising by a merchant with the inalienable right of the lone dissenter to preach his politics in the park.

Subsequently, the Court pointedly described commercial speech as enjoying only a second-class status for purposes of First Amendment analysis: "We have not discarded the common sense distinction between speech proposing a commercial transaction . . . and other varieties of speech. . . . [W]e instead have afforded commercial speech a limited measure of protection, commensurate with its subordinate position in the scale of First Amendment values. . . ." The Supreme Court knows the difference between the marketplace of products and the marketplace of ideas.

> *"Children are, in the most grisly sense of the phrase, the lifeblood of the tobacco industry."*

The high court's supportive attitude toward public regulation of advertising was judicially codified in *Central Hudson Gas & Electric Corp v Public Serv Comm'n of New York*, where, in 1980, it announced an all-purpose test for determining whether a given restriction or regulation of commercial speech violates the First Amendment. That test is still used by all state and federal courts today, and an analysis of the commonsense requirements of *Central Hudson* argues strongly in favor of the state's authority to prohibit tobacco advertising on billboards and in stores.

Central Hudson asks 4 practical questions: (1) Does the advertising serve an illegal end, or is it misleading? If so, then the advertising is not protected by the First Amendment at all. If not, the Court asks, (2) whether the governmental interest in regulating the advertising is "substantial," (3) whether that interest will be "directly advanced" by the restriction or regulation, and (4) whether the restriction or regulation is "not more extensive than is necessary to serve that interest." An affirmative answer to the latter 3 questions is required for the restriction or regulation to pass First Amendment muster.

1. Is Cigarette Advertising Misleading?

While it may be the case that tobacco advertising is inherently misleading because teenagers are moved to falsely assume that smoking is both useful and socially acceptable, Baltimore did not attempt to characterize cigarette advertising as misleading. This is appropriate because the ordinance is aimed at minimizing children's exposure to all cigarette advertising, deceptive or otherwise. Other cities or states would be well advised to follow Baltimore's example. By restricting the placement or location of tobacco advertising, rather than regulating the content or message, city administrators can avoid the complex, unending, and litigation-spawning process of examining every advertisement to determine whether it is deceptive or truthful.

Promoting the Law

2. Substantial Government Interests

The Baltimore cigarette billboard ordinance explicitly declared that its primary purpose was to help enforce a state statute that forbids the distribution of cigarettes to persons younger than 18 years. The idea is simple: By curtailing advertising that spurs the demand for cigarettes among children, state laws that seek to protect children will not be subverted.

The idea is also timely in view of the fact that the average age of smoking initiation is 14 years, addiction to smoking is almost exclusively acquired between the ages of 12 and 19 years, about 3,000 teenagers begin smoking every day, and nearly 1 billion packs of cigarettes are sold each year to persons younger than 18 years. Given that about 1.5 million adult smokers quit and another 434,000 die of smoking-related causes each year, children are, in the most grisly sense of the phrase, the lifeblood of the tobacco industry.

Not surprisingly, the district and appellate courts that reviewed Baltimore's cigarette ordinance believed that promoting observance of the state youth access law was a substantial goal for the city to pursue. The billboard company did not challenge the ordinance on that ground.

Advertising Creates Demand

3. Government Interests Directly Advanced

It would appear self-evident that a prohibition of tobacco billboard advertising would directly advance the governmental interest in promoting observance of youth access laws by reducing the demand for tobacco among young people. However, the tobacco companies and their allies contend that the $6 billion spent in 1993 on advertising and promotion of tobacco products curiously does not induce children to smoke; it only induces smokers to switch brands. According to Thomas Lauria, spokesperson for the Tobacco Institute, "There is no science behind the accusation that advertising causes smoking initiation."

No doubt the tobacco companies would be able to produce a platoon of paid expert witnesses willing to testify that there is no proven connection between tobacco advertising and aggregate demand for tobacco—as they did

> *"A prohibition of tobacco billboard advertising would directly . . . [reduce] the demand for tobacco among young people."*

in the 13-month trial challenging Canada's prohibition of all tobacco advertising, which involved 28 witnesses, 560 exhibits, and 10,819 pages of transcribed evidence. Against that testimony, a city or state could draw on the testimony of an impressive array of social scientists and a wealth of empirical data, much of it published in the *Journal of the American Medical Association*, showing that there is such a connection. The recently published findings of N. Evans and colleagues, showing that tobacco advertising is a greater influence on adolescent smoking initiation than exposure to peer or family smokers, lend considerable force to the argument, as does the 1994 *Report of the Surgeon General*, which concluded that tobacco ads do "foster the uptake of smoking."

Although such an epic battle of expert witnesses would make for good judicial theater, it is extremely unlikely that any state or local government in this country would ever have to stage such a trial. The proposition that advertising increases aggregate demand for a product, and not simply demand for a particular brand of that product, is so eminently logical that the Supreme Court and lower federal courts have repeatedly accepted it without demanding that the government provide empirical proof. In legal terms, they have taken "judicial notice" of the proposition as a "legislative fact." The Supreme Court did so in *Central Hudson* itself, in summarily finding that a New York law prohibiting advertising by electrical utilities passed the third part of the test for commercial speech regulation. The Court, even though no trial had been held and no evidence presented, agreed that there was a "connection between advertising and demand for electricity," since "Central Hudson would not contest the advertising ban unless it believed that promotion would increase its sales."

> *"Tobacco advertising is a greater influence on adolescent smoking initiation than exposure to peer or family smokers."*

Similarly, in *Posadas de Puerto Rico Associates v Tourism Co of Puerto Rico*, the Court readily accepted the Puerto Rico Legislature's belief that a ban on casino gambling advertising aimed at island residents would help curb their demand for casino gambling. To the Court, it sufficed to say that the belief was "a reasonable one."

A Reasonable Belief

Since the city of Baltimore's belief that advertising generates new consumer demand is manifestly reasonable, the city was not forced to go to trial, either in the tobacco billboard case, *Penn Advertising of Baltimore Inc v Mayor of Baltimore*, or the alcohol billboard case, *Anheuser-Busch Inc v Schmoke*. In both cases, the Fourth Circuit decided that, as a matter of law, advertising increases aggregate demand for cigarettes and alcohol, respectively. Therefore, it was not necessary to require the city to present evidence in support of those twin propositions. As the court explained in *Anheuser-Busch*:

> The City Council found that outdoor advertising is a unique and distinct medium which subjects the public to involuntary and unavoidable solicitation, and that children, simply by walking to school or playing in their neighborhood, are exposed daily to this advertising. . . . [I]t is not necessary, in satisfying *Central*

Hudson's third prong, to prove conclusively that the correlation in fact exists, or
that the steps undertaken will solve the problem [of underage drinking].

In *Penn Advertising*, the Fourth Circuit simply quoted this language to support its holding that the cigarette billboard ban also passed the third prong of the *Central Hudson* test. Accordingly, towns and states that take seriously their duty to protect children from the siren song of unavoidable outdoor tobacco advertising can look forward to rapid and relatively inexpensive judicial endorsement of a ban on such advertising.

Reasonableness

4. "Narrowly Tailored" to Achieve the Government's Objective?

In *Board of Trustees of the State University of New York v Fox*, the Supreme Court refined the fourth part of the *Central Hudson* test. The Court now asks, in its final inquiry, whether the restriction is "narrowly tailored to achieve the desired objective so as not to unduly restrict harmless speech."

In *Anheuser-Busch*, the Fourth Circuit found that the fourth prong of the *Central Hudson* test presented it with the "closest question," since the ban on alcohol billboards would deny adults, as well as children, the advertising information conveyed by that medium. However, the court also recognized that there was no "less restrictive means of screening outdoor advertising from minors," and it did not second-guess Baltimore's choice by proposing some other means of countering the pernicious effects of such advertising on children. To the contrary, it held that, "In the face of a problem as significant as that which the City seeks to address, the City must be given some reasonable latitude." The court adopted the same analysis and conclusion in *Penn Advertising*.

Baltimore acted reasonably by leaving untouched those avenues of communication that primarily reach adults and that give the consumer some control over whether to receive the message—newspapers, magazines, direct mail, and so forth. By restricting only billboard and outdoor sign advertising, which nationally accounts for only $231.5 million, or 3.8%, of the tobacco companies' total advertising and promotion budget, cities and states would leave the tobacco companies with ample alternative means to reach adults.

Sixty years ago, the Supreme Court itself recognized the reasonableness of state rules that protect the people from having cigarette ads rammed down their throats. In *Packer Corp v State of Utah*, the Court upheld Utah's complete ban on outdoor and point-of-purchase tobacco advertising against a challenge based on the Fourteenth Amendment Equal Protection Clause. The Court approvingly quoted a passage from the Utah Supreme Court's decision upholding that law:

Billboards, street car signs, and placards and such are in a class by themselves. . . . Advertisements of this sort are constantly before the eyes of observers on the streets and in street cars to be seen without the exercise of choice or volition on their part. Other forms of advertising are ordinarily seen as a matter of choice on the part of the observer. The young people as well as the adults have the message of the billboard thrust upon them by all the arts and devices that skill can produce. In the case of newspapers and magazines, there must be some seeking by the one who is to see and read the advertisement. The radio can be turned off, but not so the billboard or street car placard. These distinctions clearly place this kind of advertisement in a position to be classified so that regulations or prohibitions may be imposed upon all within the class.

Although Utah's prohibition of intrusive tobacco advertising has remained on the books for 70 years and is vigorously enforced, no one has ever challenged it again—perhaps because the Supreme Court has continued to champion the distinction between intrusive and nonintrusive speech.

In sum, a ban on outdoor tobacco advertising is a reasonable measure that deserves, and should receive, judicial approval. It does not disable any fundamental right of speech enjoyed by the tobacco giants; rather, it discharges the people's fundamental obligation to protect children from billboards that loom over them "every day while they walk to school, and every time they play in their neighborhood, thus forming an inescapable part of their daily life [*Anheuser-Busch* case].". . .

> **"A ban on outdoor tobacco advertising . . . deserves, and should receive, judicial approval."**

The capacity for billboards and other outdoor signs to inflict their messages on an unwilling audience has meant that states have been granted extraordinary authority to eliminate or control such intrusive advertising methods. In *Lehman v City of Shaker Heights*, the Supreme Court upheld a city's prohibition of political ads on its mass transit systems, in part because the advertiser "has no right to force his message upon an audience incapable of declining it."

How much stronger is a city's position when it seeks to bar from intrusive media, not political ads, but ads for a product so dangerous that its sale could be banned altogether, as the Supreme Court ruled in *Austin v Tennessee*? In fact, on the two occasions in which the Supreme Court has ruled on the constitutionality of tobacco advertising it has unanimously approved governmental restrictions on intrusive advertising methods (Utah's billboard prohibition in 1932 and Congress's ban on TV cigarette advertising in 1972). In *Posadas de Puerto Rico Associates v Tourism Co of Puerto Rico*, the high court even went so far as to rank cigarettes with such vices as gambling, alcohol, and prostitution and said that since their sale could be prohibited, their advertising could be also prohibited.

It was Justice Blackmun, the creator of the commercial speech doctrine and a vigorous defender of commercial speech, who recognized that "child pornography and cigarette advertising" will never be fully protected by the First Amendment. . . . The power of the people to protect themselves and their children from predatory cigarette advertising has never been stronger.

In sum, what these cases are saying is that it is no longer the lawyers who control the debate over tobacco advertising regulation. The legal authority states and municipalities need to at least ban tobacco ads from the most invasive media is now clearly marked, and city councils can finally get on with the business of passing ordinances instead of being frozen by fear of expensive lawsuits. The way has been made straight for physicians and public health professionals, for parents and teachers, for law officers and politicians—all citizens—to take at least a small first step toward saving the children, supporting the family, preserving the community, and upholding the law.

Chapter 4

Are Increased Measures Needed to Combat Teen Smoking?

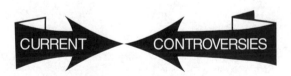

Teen Smoking and Advertising: An Overview

by Richard L. Worsnop

About the author: *Richard L. Worsnop, is an associate editor for the* CQ Researcher, *a weekly research report on public policy issues.*

Disturbed by the rise in adolescent smoking, President Clinton on Aug. 10, 1995, announced he was taking steps to counteract the trend. The action took the form of proposed FDA regulations to curb marketing of tobacco products to youths under age 18.

"When Joe Camel tells young children that smoking is cool, when billboards tell teens that smoking will lead to true romance, when Virginia Slims tell adolescents that cigarettes may make them thin and glamorous, then our children need our wisdom, our guidance and our experience," Clinton said. "We're their parents, and it is up to us to protect them."

The Proposal

The FDA proposal, issued the same day, would (1) make 18 the federal minimum age for buying tobacco products; (2) prohibit cigarette vending machines, free samples, mail-order sales and self-service displays; (3) require retailers to verify the age of young purchasers; (4) limit tobacco product ads and labels to which children are exposed to text-only "tombstone" formats; (5) bar the sale or distribution of non-tobacco promotional items bearing brand names; (6) require tobacco companies sponsoring events such as sports tournaments to identify themselves by corporate, not brand, name; and (7) make the companies establish and fund an ongoing public education campaign to discourage young people from smoking. FDA Commissioner David A. Kessler said the agency had regulatory authority over cigarettes, since they are medical "devices" under the terms of the Federal Food, Drug and Cosmetic Act.

Not surprisingly, the teen-smoking initiative won plaudits from many scientists, public health officials and anti-smoking activists. "No serious scientist

Excerpted from Richard L. Worsnop, "Teens and Tobacco," *CQ Researcher*, December 1, 1995. Reprinted with permission.

questions the fact that tobacco is the single greatest preventable cause of cancer in the United States," said National Cancer Institute Director Richard D. Klausner. He described Clinton's decision to permit FDA regulation of tobacco products as "without a doubt the most important thing in public health that he will do in his administration."

Lloyd D. Johnston, program director of the Monitoring the Future Project at the University of Michigan's Survey Research Center, also hailed the FDA proposals, saying they "would certainly move us in the right direction to reduce the amount of advertising and promotional materials that reach young people. They would remove some of the strongest stimuli that encourage adolescent smoking."

But while "reducing easy access to cigarettes is important," Johnston feels the chief value of the FDA rule package lies in "the symbolic message it sends. It says that we really do care as a society about whether our kids smoke, and that we don't want them to." He adds, "When kids have this product pushed in their face in virtually every corner of the country, it sends them another kind of message—'Tobacco must not be all that bad, because if it were, adults would protect us from it.' In fact, I've heard youngsters say exactly that."

Opposition

As was expected, cigarette makers strongly condemned the FDA's proposed rulemaking, portraying it as the first step in a campaign for prohibition of tobacco products. Indeed, Thomas Lauria, a spokesman for The Tobacco Institute, the industry's trade group, goes so far as to call the agency's action "an illegal and unconstitutional power grab" by Commissioner Kessler. "FDA hasn't got jurisdiction here," Lauria says. "They never did have jurisdiction here, and if Congress' will prevails, they'll never have jurisdiction."

In a joint motion for summary judgment filed Oct. 4, 1995 in U.S. District Court in Greensboro, N.C., the five leading cigarette manufacturers [Brown & Williamson Tobacco Corp., Liggett Group Inc., Lorillard Tobacco Co., Philip Morris Inc. and R.J. Reynolds Tobacco Co.] and a North Carolina advertising agency sought to block implementation of the FDA rules on the grounds outlined by Lauria. "On at least 20 different occasions Congress has rejected legislation that would have granted FDA jurisdiction over cigarettes," the plaintiffs declared. "On each occasion—including at least seven times over the last decade—Congress has decided that FDA should have no such authority."

> *"When Joe Camel tells young children that smoking is cool, . . . then our children need our wisdom, our guidance and our experience."*

The advertising industry, which numbers tobacco companies among its top clients, also seeks to defeat the FDA rules package in court. In a complaint filed Sept. 27, 1995, six major advertising groups [the American Advertising Federation, American Association of Advertising Agencies, Association of National Advertisers, Magazine Publishers of America, Outdoor Advertising Association of America, and Point-of-Purchase Advertising Institute] echoed some of the same arguments embodied in the cigarette makers plea to the same court. But the advertisers also contended that the FDA regulations would violate their First Amendment rights.

> *"The objective [of FDA regulations] is to reduce underage tobacco use by curtailing speech."*

"The objective of the FDA's assertion of jurisdiction over the advertising of cigarettes and smokeless tobacco products is not to create restrictions or conditions so that cigarettes and smokeless tobacco products can be used safely and effectively," the complaint stated. "The objective . . . is to reduce underage tobacco use by curtailing speech." The advertisers further charged that the FDA's move "is causing substantial irreparable injury to plaintiffs by chilling their constitutionally protected speech." Without judicial relief, "plaintiffs will face continued and lengthy uncertainty in entering into contracts and making future editorial decisions regarding advertising of tobacco products."

The Right to Advertise

Daniel L. Jaffe, executive vice president of the Association of National Advertisers, says the FDA rulemaking notice is "the most restrictive proposal in the history of this country with regard to advertising." Advertisers "have no position on whether people should smoke, or whether tobacco should be allowed to be sold or not sold," he says. "Our position is very simple: We believe that if tobacco is a legal product, which it is, it should be allowed to be advertised in a free society. That's what the First Amendment is all about. And while we agree the government should have authority to protect children, we feel it has gone way beyond that legitimate goal by trying to impose restrictions that would make it virtually impossible to advertise to anybody."

Jaffe predicts that the proposed advertising curbs "will create enormous precedents that will impact not just the tobacco companies but makers of any other controversial products," citing high-fat or high-salt foods as potential examples. He adds, "If we use children as the litmus test for what can be expressed through advertising in our society, then we are going to lower public discourse to the level of the sandbox."

The government, in Jaffe's view, is approaching the youth smoking issue from the wrong direction. "We don't stop advertising alcohol, cars or guns because they might fall into the hands of underage users," he says. "Instead, we restrict their sales. If government cracked down on illegal tobacco sales at the point of purchase, that would do more to reduce teen smoking than any conceivable restriction on advertising."

Lift the Shield

Elizabeth M. Whelan, president of the American Council on Science and Health, a consumer advocacy group in New York, devotes much of her time to what she calls the "cigarette tragedy." But as a conservative Republican, she feels the proposed FDA regulations are misconceived and heavyhanded. In her view, the best way to discourage smoking within all age groups is to make to-bacco companies play by the same liability rules as other industries. The best way to do this, she says, is to have Congress remove the government-mandated warning labels from cigarette packs.

"[A]s a result of the label, tobacco-company lawyers have consistently and successfully argued in court that Congress has pre-empted their responsibility for warning consumers about any diseases that cigarettes might cause," Whelan noted. "If we were truly serious about confronting an industry that is literally selling death, we would remove the government warning label and thus strip the tobacco industry of this privileged legal status."

If the shield were lifted, Whelan says, the tobacco industry itself would have to inform consumers in detail about the health consequences of smoking. That would mean, in turn, that warning labels on cigarette packs "would be about the size of the New York City phone book.". . .

Teen Smoking Trends

The percentage of high school seniors smoking at least one cigarette a day slid from 28.9 percent in 1977 to 17.2 percent in 1992, according to data gath-ered by the University of Michigan's Monitoring the Future Project. The drop was even sharper among black youngsters, a trend that intrigues researchers on both sides of the smoking issue. Many experts attributed the teen-smoking de-cline to the disappearance of broadcast cigarette commercials [in 1970].

That theory seemed less persuasive after the Monitoring the Future Project re-ported that 19.4 percent of high school seniors were smokers in 1994. One rea-son for the turnaround, Johnston suggested, is that teens "greatly overestimate their ability to stop smoking once they have begun, so they are making deci-sions about whether or not to smoke at a very early age, with little or no appreciation of the likely conse-quences of those decisions."

> *"[Teens] are making decisions about whether or not to smoke at a very early age."*

Patrick M. O'Malley, a colleague of Johnston's, noted that even two years of increased smoking by teens will have lasting consequences. "We know that once a birth cohort establishes a particularly high or low rate of smoking in adolescence, relative to other birth cohorts, it continues to maintain a relatively high or low rate throughout the life cycle," he said. "Thus the higher rates that we are observing now are likely to remain high later in life for these children."

Johnston foresees no "immediate reversal" of the current trend. "It's a little like the proverbial battleship," he says. "It'll take time to make it change direction. Also, we have to realize that kids entering the age groups we survey have already been subjected to years of persuasion by the tobacco industry."

Whelan has first-hand knowledge of smoking patterns among high school seniors. "My daughter just graduated from a private girls school here in New York, and half of the 32 seniors smoked," she says. "I felt a sense of defeat, because these young women had been warned about the dangers of cigarettes since kindergarten. And even so, they smoke. What can I say?"

Whelan acknowledges that the insistent warnings of anti-smoking activists may backfire among teenagers, who often resent adult authority figures. "My daughter once said to me, 'If I hear one more thing about smoking, maybe I should try it. There must be something great about cigarettes if you keep talking about them that much.'"

Increased Measures Are Needed to Combat Teen Smoking

by Randolph D. Smoak Jr.

About the author: *Randolph D. Smoak Jr. is a trustee for the American Medical Association, the primary professional association of physicians in the United States.*

Editor's note: The following text is excerpted from a speech delivered to the Tobacco Liability Project on November 10, 1995.

I have had many proud moments as a physician. However, one of my proudest moments as a public health advocate was August 10, 1995, when the FDA [Food and Drug Administration] and President Bill Clinton announced their regulations to stop wholesale addiction of our children. Children are fodder to the tobacco industry. Each year, they must lure more than 400,000 children to begin smoking to replace those who die annually of heart, lung and cancerous ailments. Sadly, they are succeeding. Between 1991 and 1995, the number of eighth graders who smoke has risen 30 percent. Eighth grade—that's 13 years old. So today, I stand here on behalf of my new granddaughter born just 16 days ago—to say no more addiction and no more targeting of children.

The fight against tobacco cannot be a single front battle. The tobacco industry is so well established and fortified that only the combined efforts of literally thousands of advocates can realistically stop the epidemic of tobacco-caused disease in this country—and for that matter the world.

Four Avenues

There are four avenues we must pursue to control tobacco:

First—public health programs. A significant minority of the public still do not link tobacco use with lung cancer, heart disease, or chronic lung diseases.

From Randolph D. Smoak Jr., "The AMA's Tobacco Fight," a speech delivered to the Tobacco Liability Project, Boston, Mass., November 10, 1995. Reprinted by permission.

And teens don't think they will die from ANY risky behavior. If we do not continue and increase our education of potential new smokers, then we are partially responsible for their addiction.

Second—anti-tobacco advertising and public perception campaigns.

Unless we pursue, educate, and attempt to influence youth attitudes and perceptions of tobacco by de-normalizing tobacco use and isolating the tobacco companies, showing them to be a rogue industry—then we will not overcome the $6 billion spent annually in tobacco advertising that helps to addict our children.

Again, the evidence is overwhelming that advertising is a key reason teenagers begin smoking. On October 14, 1995, a study in the *Journal of the National Cancer Institute*, an esteemed, peer-viewed journal, clearly showed that youth are more heavily influenced by advertising than peer pressure. There is almost nothing more powerful to teens than peer pressure, but now we understand the other, more powerful force, fed by the tobacco industry. That is tobacco advertising.

Government Regulation

Number three, we must use prudent government intervention and regulation.

An industry—any industry—that wantonly disregards the health and welfare of its customers and shows no signs of reforming its manner of conducting business must be regulated by government.

Personally, I find it unbelievable that many argue the FDA has no legal standing to regulate tobacco consumption. The FDA can regulate aspirin, "twinkies" and orange juice—but not tobacco? What sense does that make?

Regarding tobacco advertising, for example, regulations proposed by the FDA would bar several kinds of tobacco advertising and promotion, including the attractive "Marlboro Gear" and "Camel Cash" campaigns that create walking cigarette ads with brand-name clothing that kids like so much. And several local communities, the city of Baltimore, for instance, have banned tobacco billboards and other local advertising. The FDA also proposes a national "counter-advertising" campaign funded by the tobacco industry.

> *"Regulations [on tobacco advertising] . . . have the possibility of significantly reducing the number of adolescents hooked each year."*

We think the FDA regulations announced by the President have the possibility of significantly reducing the number of adolescents hooked each year—in most cases many years prior to their 18th birthday.

Prudent regulation is necessary. . . . Local laws have cleared many workplaces, restaurants and other public areas. Local and state laws also regulate the sale of tobacco products to minors, rules that are enforced in the breach, for the most part. The industry, despite its protests that it doesn't want kids as customers, continues to subvert these laws by attempting to make it illegal to sell tobacco to children, for example, only if the merchant does so knowingly and willingly. You must be willing to play a leadership role in enforcing meaningful laws that keep tobacco out of the hands of children, and must not fall for the Trojan Horse compromises offered by tobacco lobbyists.

Fourth, any industry that kills 400,000 of its best customers each year must be held accountable—socially and economically—for the enormous cost it extracts with a proven, deadly product.

The AMA agrees that it is important to hold these tobacco merchants accountable through your work in the courtrooms of America and, using the power of your offices to enforce tobacco controls, provide consumer—and I must add "child"—protection and defend those local governments under attack from tobacco representatives for anti-smoking laws. In West Virginia, tobacco lawyers are suing local Boards of Health in an attempt to keep them from protecting the public from the health hazards of indoor tobacco smoke pollution. Several communities are under attack for daring to propose local advertising restrictions or ban vending machines. They need your help.

None of these four areas are more important than the others. They are the four legs of a table. Without aggressively pursuing each of the four, the table will crash to the floor and all our hopes and aspirations for a healthier tomorrow will be gone. . . .

A Doctor's Story

Let me finish today with my story. I am a general surgeon. I have removed cancerous lungs. I have removed cancer of the throat, larynx and voice box, tongue, jaw and gums of hundreds of patients whose faces I will never forget. I have watched the tears roll down the faces of my patients and their families as I have told them of their cancer. I have heard their words of regret for not overcoming their addiction to tobacco. So, I must tell you I had great difficulty one year ago watching seven leaders of the tobacco industry raise their hands and swear before this nation and God that they do not believe nicotine is addictive.

Who knows, they may honestly believe that. But I have raised my right hand with a scalpel too often not to know—they are dead wrong.

In South Carolina—tobacco country—where I practice, chewing tobacco is still very popular. In fact, its use is growing. Kids walk with the perfect circle of a chew can in the back pocket of their fading blue jeans. I've operated on a bunch of these great kids later in their life—some when they are in their 20's or 30's. And I can tell exactly what part of the Carolinas they are from without even glancing at their chart. In a certain number of counties, they chew here on the side and back. Other counties they place the chew up front here between the teeth and front lip. And so on. Wherever they place their chew— that's where I'll find the cancer. I know nicotine is addictive. I know, firsthand, it causes terrible, terrible cancer.

Increased Government Regulations Are Necessary to Reduce Teen Smoking

by Henry Waxman

About the author: *Henry Waxman is the Democratic representative of California's Twenty-fourth Congressional District. He serves on the Energy and Commerce, Government Operations, and Select Aging Committees. He has long been a strong supporter of antismoking legislation.*

Every year, some of the world's most powerful corporations hook millions of American children on a drug that is as addictive as heroin or cocaine—and far more deadly than either. Unless we act now, many of these children will die from their addiction decades from now.

The drug is nicotine. And the corporations are America's tobacco companies.

The Costs of Smoking

The tobacco companies market image but the cold statistics show that cigarettes kill nearly half a million Americans every year. The annual cost to our health-care system is tens of billions of dollars in preventable expenses.

The tobacco companies' success—and the sickness and death that result—starts with kids. The companies spend billions on advertising campaigns that entice young teen-agers to smoke. Each year hundreds of thousands of teen-agers become lifelong addicts, destined to die of lung cancer, heart disease and other tobacco-related causes.

Even those kids who reject cigarettes are not safe. Their health is threatened by exposure to other people's tobacco smoke.

Despite the overwhelming evidence of the risks of smoking, the tobacco companies have been chillingly effective in stopping proposals to regulate the use of tobacco. It's time to fight back. Four simple measures would protect all of us, especially our children:

Henry Waxman, "Stop the Drugging of Our Children," *Los Angeles Times*, April 11, 1994. Reprinted with permission.

The first and easiest step is a law requiring smoke-free public areas and workplaces. . . .

Enactment of such legislation . . . would produce enormous benefits at minimal cost. Nonsmoking people would be protected from carcinogenic tobacco smoke. Hundreds of thousands of asthmatic children could go to restaurants, bowling alleys and other public places without fear of a life-threatening attack. And building owners would save billions by avoiding the costs of cleaning up cigarette smoke and ashes. Even smokers would benefit, because quitting is much easier in smoke-free environments.

According to the federal Environmental Protection Agency, compliance with a national smoke-free policy in public and workplaces would, each year, save 38,000 to 108,000 lives and produce $11.5 billion to $29 billion in medical and economic savings—all for a cost of less than $1 billion annually.

The next two steps are to raise the tax on tobacco and to restrict cigarette advertising. These measures share a common goal: to protect health by reducing the consumption of cigarettes. According to some estimates, increasing the tax on a pack of cigarettes by $2 could reduce tobacco use by 23%, eventually save the lives of 2 million Americans and raise more than $23 billion each year for health-care reform.

The advertising restrictions are particularly important for children, who are the targets of cigarette ad campaigns featuring "Joe Camel" and Marlboro's "Adventure Team." The Tobacco Education and Child Protection Act, which I introduced, would stop the tobacco industry's most abusive tactics, such as advertising and distributing free samples near schools. New and bigger warning labels would also be required on all advertisements.

The last reform is to get nicotine out of cigarettes. Among adult smokers, 70% say they would quit if they could. Removing addictive nicotine from cigarettes would allow these smokers to choose for themselves whether to continue to smoke.

For children especially, nicotine-free cigarettes would be a literal lifesaver. If there were no nicotine, youthful experimentation with cigarettes would not lead to addiction.

These four reforms—all overdue—would end the special treatment tobacco companies receive from the federal government. And they may now be possible. Public sentiment is surging against the tobacco companies as never before. Almost daily another company or state or local government announces new restrictions on smoking. Indeed, Congress passed legislation to ban smoking in schools, day-care centers and medical clinics that receive federal funding.

We must face a reality too long ignored and finally take decisive action against tobacco. Nothing less than the lives of hundreds of thousands of our children are at stake.

Antismoking Ads Can Persuade Teens Not to Smoke

by Yumiko Ono

About the author: *Yumiko Ono is a staff reporter for the* Wall Street Journal.

"Smoking Stinks," declares a California billboard with a ponytailed teenage girl gagging as her boyfriend blows cigarette smoke into her face.

To 14-year-old Charles Eisenmann, viewing a slide of the billboard, it's the ad that stinks. "If she doesn't like it, she should just get away from him," says Charles, a ninth-grader from Kansas City, Mo., and a member of the city's Red Bridge YMCA Adventure Club, which recently convened a group of teenagers to talk about antismoking ads.

Far more effective, Charles says, is an ad featuring baseball and football star Deion Sanders, scowling, with the message: "The only things I smoke are pitchers, catchers, quarterbacks and receivers." Charles, who started smoking two years ago, says the Sanders ad encouraged him to quit. . . .

As Charles's experience suggests, when it comes to smoking and kids, it's hard to figure out which ads miss the mark and which hit home.

No One Message

"When something is as much a part of your culture as smoking, there is no one [message] that stops it," says Colleen Stevens, chief of the tobacco media unit at the California Department of Health Services. Her office has used state cigarette excise taxes to fund an antismoking ad campaign. Not only does California vary the content of its youth-oriented antismoking messages, it also airs them in Mandarin, Cantonese and Spanish, as well as English. In 1994, the state spent $12 million on the print and broadcast campaign.

Although some campaigns around the country have focused on real-life, smoking-induced catastrophic illnesses and deaths, many avoid health warnings aimed at youths. "Kids think they will live forever. Talking about a disease you may get when you're 50 or 60 isn't a compelling motivator," says Lisa Unsworth, executive vice president at Houston Effler Herstek Favat. The Boston ad agency has created ads since 1993 for Massachusetts, which, like California, uses cigarette taxes to pay for the campaign.

Instead, Houston Effler plays up more immediate consequences, such as performing badly in sports. One commercial shows an agile nonsmoker beating wheezing smokers in a basketball game. "If you smoke, you can't breathe. If you can't breathe, you can't run. If you can't run, you can't win," says the grinning youth, as his smoking competitor slides haplessly across the floor.

The message scores with 12-year-old Kalinda Franklin of the Adventure Club group. "It's true!" she says with a giggle. "When you play basketball, they try to mess you up, and if you smoke, you can't play well." But Matt Welliver, another club member, isn't convinced. "That's for people who smoke a pack in 15 minutes," says the 14-year-old.

One common piece of advice from antismoking advertisers: Avoid making cigarettes appear to be "forbidden fruit." Some advertisers criticize a poster Philip Morris Cos. sends stores, warning: "If you ask for cigarettes, we ask for I.D." "It's like saying, 'You can't do this, you're not old enough,'" says Joseph Cherner, president of SmokeFree Educational Services Inc., a New York-based nonprofit health-advocacy group. "It just provokes the reaction, oh yeah? I'll show you."

Philip Morris says the poster is aimed mainly at sales clerks, to remind them not to sell to minors.

> *"It's hard to figure out which ads miss the mark and which hit home."*

More broadly, says spokeswoman Ellen Merlo, teenagers "tend to say that advertising doesn't cause them to start smoking, and it's not going to cause them to stop smoking."

Study Shows Ads Work

Nevertheless, a 1992 study by the University of Vermont suggests antismoking ads may indeed have an impact on the young. The study tracked the smoking initiation rates of 5,458 students in grades four through six for four years. Researchers blitzed one pair of communities with 10 antismoking TV ads a week and left another pair of communities without any ads. The result: Questionnaires given to the participants during the course of the study showed that the percentage of kids who smoked in the week prior to the questionnaire was 35% lower in communities with the ads than in those without them.

As for campaign themes, the Adventure Club discussion shows that the use of humor in antismoking messages can be effective but poses problems. Michelle McKinney, a 13-year-old club member with braided hair and a denim beret, scoffs at an American Lung Association poster featuring Brooke Shields with cigarettes sticking out of her ears. "Smoking spoils your looks" is the tagline.

"Why is it coming out of her ears, and not her mouth?" Michelle asks.

Still, humor—particularly of the macabre variety—can sometimes help point up smoking's hazards. SmokeFree, the New York nonprofit, held an anti-smoking-poster contest for New York City kids and displayed the winners as subway ads. One, created by a fifth-grader, shows a picture of a skeleton with a cowboy hat, riding a horse into a cemetery. The caption: "Come to where the cancer is." The poster was so popular that more than 15,000 of them were stolen since 1990, says SmokeFree's Mr. Cherner.

Another SmokeFree winner, made by a 12th-grader, shows a wrinkled woman grinning through her brownish-yellow teeth and holding a cigarette with her stained fingers. "Virginia Slime— You've Come the Wrong Way, Baby," says the headline.

> *"Antismoking ads may indeed have an impact on the young."*

Some themes that adults reject as too corny may click for kids. Jane Rinzler, who surveyed hundreds of kids for Houston Effler's Massachusetts ads, proposed pushing the idea that smoking is a bad influence on younger siblings. "I kept going back to the agency, and they said, 'Come on, you're kidding,'" Ms. Rinzler says. But she persisted, and Houston Efner filmed a commercial featuring a serious-looking teenage boy looking on at scenes of frolicking preschoolers. "If we smoke, they will smoke," the teenager warns.

Bill Wortman, 12, who goes to the Adventure Club with his 14-year-old brother, Jim, doesn't buy the message and insists he won't start smoking even if Jim does. But the rest of the group immediately erupts with shrieks of derision. "That's the first thing you're going to do, Bill!" screams one, as Bill blushes and falls silent.

"It's probably true," reflects Jim Wortman later. "If I do something, my brother's going to follow my footsteps."

Peer Groups Can Help Keep Teens from Smoking

by Sara Rimer

About the author: *Sara Rimer is a reporter for the* New York Times *newspaper.*

Priscilla Purvis was outraged when she saw a small boy buy a single cigarette at a convenience store in her inner-city neighborhood not long ago.

"He said, 'Can I get a "loosie"?'" recalled Priscilla, 16, who has never smoked a cigarette and vows she never will. "He paid 15 cents for it and left. He was about 9 years old. I just went totally off on the store owner. I said, 'He's a little boy—that's illegal.'"

Priscilla, who says she hopes never to catch her 11-year-old brother with a cigarette, added, "Now I'm thinking I should've gone after the boy."

Three million Americans under the age of 18 smoke, according to the United States Surgeon General's office, and every day 3,000 minors have their first cigarettes. Surgeon General studies have also shown that 82 percent of the people who smoke began before their 18th birthday, suggesting that anyone who does not smoke before adulthood might be unlikely to ever begin.

Antismoking Soldiers

Despite a surge in teen-age smoking, there are still plenty of young people, like Priscilla Purvis, who consider the habit a dangerous addiction and the antithesis of cool—and who have become soldiers in a growing antismoking youth movement. While Priscilla is part of an effort organized and financed by the Massachusetts Department of Public Health, other states have begun similar, though smaller, programs.

"I talk to teen-agers all the time," said Priscilla, a peer leader in a state-supported program at the Dimock Community Health Center in her Roxbury neighborhood. "They say, 'Oh, I'm so stressed out, that's why I smoke.' I tell them, 'You want to fit in with everyone else, that's why you smoke. Little do you know, none of you look cool.' I tell them, 'You stink, and you don't look good.'"

The program, part of a broader state effort to combat smoking by people of all ages, has drawn Federal attention and helped make Massachusetts a model for programs to counteract the youth-oriented marketing of the tobacco industry.

For example, state workers and volunteers set up booths at 11 Massachusetts malls and persuaded 25,000 teen-agers to join a movement for a smoke-free generation. In return, the teen-agers received discounts of 10 to 15 percent at 150 stores offering incentives.

The state's drive to crack down on merchants who sell cigarettes to minors has had a measurable effect, officials say. In a sting operation, the state found that only 28 percent of the cigarette outlets surveyed would readily sell to people under 18, down from the 70 percent found in a sting 18 months earlier. More broadly, officials say total cigarette sales have fallen 15 percent.

> *"There are still plenty of young people . . . who consider the habit a dangerous addiction and the antithesis of cool."*

There is, of course, a price for such results. For two years, Massachusetts spent $36 million a year on its anti-smoking campaign, "It's Time We Make Smoking History," more than any other state except California. Most of the money is raised by a 25-cents-per-pack cigarette tax approved by the voters in 1992 after a strong push by the Massachusetts division of the American Cancer Society.

About $14 million is spent on television advertising primarily directed at teen-agers, said Dr. Greg Connolly, the director of the health department's Tobacco Control Program. Much of the balance, he said, is used to train, organize and supervise antismoking youth groups like Priscilla's at the Dimock Center, to mount efforts like mall petition drives and to press communities to enact tougher regulations—and then enforce them—against selling tobacco products to minors. So far, 132 local governments have done so in Massachusetts.

A Hard-Hitting Effort

The Food and Drug Administration said the antismoking program in Massachusetts, as well as one in California, had helped pave the way toward tough antismoking regulations and policies endorsed by President Clinton with the aim of keeping tobacco away from young people.

"Massachusetts is an especially good example of a hard-hitting educational effort that tells kids the truth about tobacco," said Jim O'Hara, a spokesman for the F.D.A.

Dr. Connolly said, "We do know we've reduced the ability of teen-agers to buy cigarettes."

But the pressures on young people to smoke are enormous. A survey of 1,200 teen-agers by Dr. Connolly's office found that 21 percent had a T-shirt or hat with a tobacco company logo. Teen-agers get these and similar brand-oriented items with the cigarettes they buy or by mailing in coupons from cigarette packages. Sherina Hendrix, 15, a peer leader from Boston's Dorchester neighborhood, said that red leather Marlboro jackets were popular now at her school.

Dr. Connolly said the program's antismoking television commercials played down the role of the Public Health Department. "Kids don't like the government telling them what to do," he explained.

> *"Recruiting and training young people to counsel others on the dangers of smoking . . . was crucial."*

At the same time, he added, the commercials, as well as the peer training, try to show young people that they are being manipulated by a tobacco industry that portrays smoking as glamorous.

Luis Reyes, 15, a peer leader at the Dimock Health Center, has the message. "When they're advertising cigarettes," he said, "showing those people with their white teeth, skinny, all happy, they don't tell the truth."

Dr. Connolly said that recruiting and training young people to counsel others on the dangers of smoking, a technique called peer counseling, was crucial. "They're our shock troops," he said. "They put out the message that smoking is not cool. It's not adults talking down to kids."

Rosa DePina, 17, of Boston, said her training to become a peer counselor had persuaded her not to smoke. "I thought cigarettes had no effect at all," she said. "All my friends smoke. Everyone in my family smokes. Even the ones who are pretty old—like in their 40's—smoke, and they seem O.K."

Yet Rosa still buys loosies at the corner store for her 21-year-old brother when he asks. "That's my brother," she said. "I have to. He does not listen to me."

In fact, many teen-agers do not like being told what to do, or not do, by anyone, no matter their age or relationship. "He gets on my nerves," said Dennis Toran, 16, who smokes a pack of Marlboro Lights a day, referring to Tim Rogers, a friend and peer leader in their South Boston neighborhood. "He won't stop nagging me. He crushes my cigarettes and stuff."

Tim, 15, who likes to stay healthy so he can excel at basketball, football and hockey, said, "I can't see why anyone would want smoke coming into their bodies."

Buying Loosies

Priscilla and her 600 fellow peer leaders statewide, who are paid $6 an hour for their part-time work, do more than just talk about the evils of smoking to other youngsters. In Roxbury and other inner-city neighborhoods, they have visited dozens of stores, asking the owners to sign pledges agreeing not to sell minors single-cigarette loosies or any cigarettes.

Another peer leader at the Dimock Center in Roxbury, Calvin Langford, 15, declared: "I feel it should be canceled completely, the whole tobacco industry. There are kids younger than me who smoke who can't even run up and down the basketball court without getting out of breath."

The idea of trying to stop sales of loosies came from Michele Williams, a program coordinator at Women Inc., a residential substance abuse treatment center. "I hate loosies," Ms. Williams said. "I've never seen a kid buy a pack of cigarettes. But I've seen them buy loosies all the time. That's how they get started."

In Chicopee, in western Massachusetts, a group of teen-agers operating under the auspices of the state program waged a successful campaign to get the one mall in the city to declare itself smoke-free.

"Smoking is gross," said one member of the group, Jeannie Stokowski, 15. "It turns me off. If I ever see a guy smoking, I'm not interested. I would never kiss a guy who smoked. It would put me in danger because of secondhand smoke."

In 1993 in Gloucester, a fishing village 30 miles north of Boston, four seventh-grade girls collected enough petition signatures to persuade the City Council to ban most cigarette vending machines in public places.

"We thought, 'Oh, God, we have the vending-machine owners here,'" said one of the girls, Alicia Cox, 14, recalling the meeting at which the council voted unanimously for the ban. "We got up and said, 'Would you rather have business or save lives?' They didn't have anything to say after that."

In the South Boston neighborhood, peer leaders recently got the South Boston Boys and Girls Club to forbid anyone to bring cigarettes into the club.

"We were trying to prove that cigarettes are a drug, just like alcohol," Tim Rogers said.

Another South Boston peer leader, 16-year-old Audrey Gobiel, said she felt no social pressure to smoke. "I don't need to smoke to be cool," she said. "I'm my own person. I think of myself as cool for what I am."

The Seriousness of the Teen Smoking Problem Is Exaggerated

by Michelle Maglalang Malkin

About the author: *Michelle Maglalang Malkin was the 1995 Warren Brookes fellow at the Competitive Enterprise Institute, an organization that advocates free enterprise. She is currently on staff at the* Seattle Times.

In one of countless anti-smoking missives, Jimmy Carter warned: "We must not be tricked again." This is an apt, if unintended, admonition. For the Clinton administration's 1995 regulatory offensive—backed blindly by Jimmy Carter, Barry Goldwater and a broad coalition of anti-tobacco organizations—was not an honest effort to rescue America's youth from the perils of puffing. It was yet another thinly-disguised attempt to puff up the federal government's public health powers by creating a phantom childhood epidemic.

President Clinton cited an alarming rise in pre-teen and teen-age smoking as the impetus for his initiative: "The most important thing is that there is an epidemic among our children." Mr. Clinton's health mandarins echoed the sentiment. Food and Drug Commissioner David Kessler, whose power will swell under the new plan, spoke of a "pediatric disease." Health and Human Services Secretary Donna Shalala lamented that attempts to reduce underage smoking have failed. And Michael Eriksen, director of the Surgeon General's Office on Smoking and Health at the Centers for Disease Control and Prevention proclaimed: "There is absolutely no question that teen smoking rates are on the rise. The only people who are denying this are spokespersons for the tobacco industry."

Is There an Epidemic?

But is there an epidemic? Tobacco flacks aren't the only ones who are questioning the administration's allegations. Anyone who has diagnosed the White House's bad habit of using children to justify federal power grabs (recall the

Michelle Maglalang Malkin, "The Epidemic That Isn't," *Washington Times*, August 14, 1995. Reprinted with permission.

vaccine warehouse fiasco?) knows better than to accept manufactured claims of childhood health epidemics on faith alone.

The most-oft cited data on youth smoking comes from the University of Michigan's Monitoring the Future project, a federally funded study initiated 20 years ago. In 1995, university researchers released highly-publicized statistics showing incremental increases in lifetime, daily and occasional (one or more cigarettes over a 30-day period) use by eighth-, 10th- and 12th-graders. From 1991 to 1994, lifetime use among eighth-graders (the youngest group surveyed) increased from 44 percent to 46.1 percent; occasional use, 14.3 percent to 18.6 percent; and daily use, 7.2 to 8.8 percent. Press reports latched onto these numbers in particular to proclaim a "surge," "huge jump," and "alarming rise" in cigarette use by children.

That there has been a small increase in pre-teen smoking since 1991 is irrefutable. We should be worried, no question. But what the White House and the media failed to emphasize, however, is that the survey only began monitoring eighth-graders and 10th-graders in 1991. Statistical trends for these groups are but a small subset of a larger data series that dates back to 1975. A look at the big picture, undistorted by selective statistical gerrymandering, shows promising downward trends. Overall, daily smoking among high school seniors has been steadily declining. (See chart.) Moreover heavy smoking by the nation's 12th-graders (a half-pack a day or more) plunged from 17.9 percent in 1975 to 11.2 percent in 1984, remaining flat for the subsequent decade.

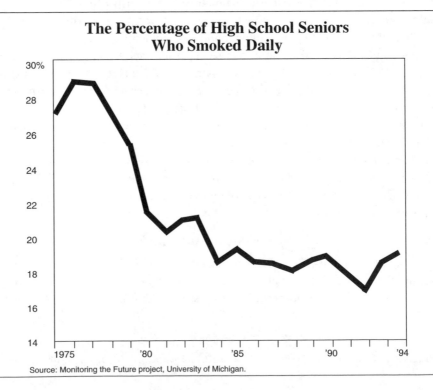

The Percentage of High School Seniors Who Smoked Daily

Source: Monitoring the Future project, University of Michigan.

Blacks and Smoking

Another astonishing phenomenon buried by the White House hoopla: the great decline in smoking by black teens. In 1980, 25.2 percent of black high school seniors smoked at least one cigarette over the past 30 days; by 1994, the figure had dropped to 11.0 percent—no thanks to President Clinton, the Food and Drug Administration or the tobacco industry.

Finally, the Michigan study offers data on a far more dramatic rise in recent years—the increase in marijuana use by pre-teens and teens of both races and sexes. After dropping steadily for the past decades, occasional use among high school seniors spiked from 11.9 percent in 1992 to 19 percent in 1994; among all eighth-graders, use more than doubled, from 3.2 percent to 7.8 percent from 1991 to 1994. So should we expect an anti-marijuana initiative from our non-inhaling president anytime soon? Don't hold your breath.

Current Antismoking Measures Aimed at Teens Are Sufficient

by J. Howard Beales

About the author: *J. Howard Beales is an associate professor of strategic management and public policy at George Washington University in Washington, D.C.*

Teenage smoking provokes controversy and continuing policy proposals to "do something" about a phenomenon that all would prefer did not exist. From the rhetoric surrounding the issue, a casual observer would likely conclude that teen smoking was either a recent problem or a rapidly increasing one. Neither perception is correct, despite recent reports of an increase in smoking among high school students. Although teenage smoking remains a concern, the facts suggest that the long-standing policy of educating teens as well as adults about the risks of smoking is working and is resulting in significant declines in smoking.

The Extent of Teenage Smoking

The most recent large-scale national study of teenage smoking available is the Teenage Attitudes and Practices Survey (TAPS), conducted by the Centers for Disease Control in 1989. The survey reveals that just over two-thirds of 11- to 17-year-old teens—who cannot legally smoke in most states—have not smoked even one whole cigarette. Even among 17-year-olds, a majority have not yet smoked a cigarette.

Teens who have experimented with cigarettes are considered smokers by the standard government definition if they have smoked one cigarette in the previous 30 days. By that definition, 13 percent of 11- to 17-year-olds were smokers. There are significant differences between younger and older teens. Although only 1 percent of 11-year-olds have smoked in the previous 30 days, 24 percent of 17-year-olds have done so, as have 31 percent of 18- and 19-year-olds. Thus,

J. Howard Beales, "Teenage Smoking: Fact and Fiction," *American Enterprise*, March/April 1994. Reprinted by permission of the *American Enterprise*, a Washington-based magazine of politics, business, and culture.

most teenage smokers are older teens. Furthermore, most teenage smokers are social smokers, who smoke only occasionally, rather than daily smokers. Although some 60 percent of young adult (18- to 24-year-old) smokers are daily smokers, only about a third of teenage smokers smoke daily.

The standard definition of a teenage smoker as someone who has smoked one cigarette in the previous 30 days lumps together teens who are serious smokers and those who are recent experimenters. In fact, 27 percent of the teens defined as smokers used cigarettes on 4 or fewer days during the previous month. Obviously, some teens that researchers classify as smokers do not consider themselves smokers and do not smoke to any significant extent.

Among adults, researchers generally avoid the problem by asking whether respondents consider themselves smokers. The effect of the difference in definitions is to overstate teenage smoking relative to adult smoking. Indeed, about 22 percent of young adults in California (where such a comparison was made) who would be considered smokers under the definition used for teens are not smokers under the standard adult definition.

> *"The long-standing policy of educating teens . . . about the risks of smoking is working."*

Appreciating the difference between having tried a cigarette and being a smoker is necessary in order to understand the age at which teens begin to smoke. Among 11- to 17-year-old teens who have smoked a cigarette, the median age of the first cigarette was 13. This median age is undoubtedly lower than it would have been if all teenagers had been questioned. Moreover, most teens have never smoked a cigarette. Thus, only about 18 percent of 11- to 17-year-olds have tried a cigarette by age 13. Additionally, many, and perhaps most, of those who try a cigarette will never become regular smokers. A California study found that among young adults (ages 18–24), a majority of those who have tried cigarettes have *never* smoked regularly. Even among those who have at one time been regular smokers, the median age at which they first smoked regularly was 16.

Trends

Few reliable statistics are available to track the incidence of teen smoking over time. Government studies of teens as a group have been sporadic. The most consistent data available are from an annual survey of high school seniors conducted by researchers at the University of Michigan since 1975.

Cigarette use among high school seniors peaked in 1976. Whether measured as smoking in the past 30 days, daily smoking, or smoking half a pack a day, smoking had declined 20 to 25 percent from that peak by 1980. Since then, the decline in smoking has been less rapid. Moreover, all three measures show an increase in 1993.

If one examines the incidence of smoking in the previous 30 days, teenage smoking since 1980 has been roughly constant, with a slight downward drift through 1992. Counting those who have smoked in the previous 30 days, however, measures both real smokers and teens who have recently experimented with cigarettes, perhaps for the first time. Indeed, success in encouraging younger teens to delay experimenting with cigarettes could actually increase the incidence of recent smoking among high school seniors. Measures of the incidence of daily smoking and smoking half a pack a day are less prone to this problem. These measures, which fell about 25 percent between 1976 and 1980, showed continued declines throughout the 1980s. By 1993, daily smoking was down 11 percent from 1980, and smoking half a pack a day was down 24 percent. Thus, measures of significant cigarette use show continued declines, albeit at a less rapid rate than during the late 1970s. The fraction of high school seniors who have ever smoked even one cigarette, which declined only 6 percent by 1980, also continued to decline, falling an additional 13 percent by 1992.

Some have argued that the apparent increases in smoking in 1993 mark the beginning of a new and worrisome trend. Although definitive answers must await additional surveys, it seems more likely that the 1993 results simply reflect chance variations from year to year. The increases, after all, were from the lowest levels of smoking that the survey had ever recorded. The fraction of high school seniors who have ever smoked a cigarette was virtually unchanged, increasing by only a tenth of a percentage point. Moreover, preliminary data from a 1993 follow-up of the earlier TAPS study indicate that smoking by 15- to 17-year-old teens had declined. Certainly, the 1993 uptick provides no basis for aggressive new policies aimed at teenage smoking.

To the extent that the smoking increases are real, they appear to reflect an increased willingness of teens to engage in a variety of risky behaviors. Indeed, the survey found substantially larger increases in the use of illegal drugs, particularly marijuana (up 30 percent based on use in the past 30 days) and hallucinogens (up 28 percent), than in the use of cigarettes (up 7.6 percent).

Why Do Teens Smoke?

Many discussions of public policy toward teenage smoking presume that teenage smoking decisions are fundamentally irrational. Implicitly or explicitly, teenage smokers are treated as the passive victims of social forces compelling

> *"Most teenage smokers are social smokers."*

them to smoke, forces that are utterly beyond their control. In sharp contrast, careful statistical analysis of actual smoking behavior indicates that teenagers' decisions are, in an economic sense, rational: teens assess the expected benefits and costs of smoking and make their decisions accordingly.

Using data on the characteristics of teens who smoke at different levels of intensity (for example, daily smokers versus occasional smokers versus those who have tried cigarettes but are not current smokers), statistical analysis can disentangle the various influences on teenage smoking decisions. Essentially, the statistical analysis determines which factors best account for the observed smoking behavior of teens.

Three sets of factors are important influences on teenage smoking. Most important is the behavior of their peers. Teens whose friends are smokers are significantly more likely to be smokers themselves. Second, teen perceptions of the risks of smoking, along with perceptions of benefits such as helping to relax or combat stress, are important determinants of behavior. Finally, the presence of smokers in teen households influences smoking decisions.

> *"Teens substantially overestimate the risk of smoking."*

One way to compare the relative importance of different influences on the smoking decision is to determine the likelihood that a teen with a particular set of characteristics will have smoked in the previous 30 days. As a base case, consider a 15-year-old from a family of average income who is white, non-Hispanic, and goes out two or three nights per week for recreation. Like most teens, this baseline teen has uniformly negative attitudes about smoking—he or she thinks that even an occasional cigarette is harmful, that smoking for a year or two is dangerous, and that smoking offers no benefits. None of his or her family members or friends are smokers. For this hypothetical teen, the likelihood of smoking is 1.85 percent. That is, just under 2 percent of teens with these characteristics should be smokers. (For comparison, about 16 percent of 15-year-olds in the sample actually were smokers.) We can then assess the importance of changing any of these factors by determining the change in the likelihood of smoking compared to this baseline teen. If, for example, a particular factor doubles the base probability of smoking to 3.7 percent, the relative odds for that factor would be 2. . . .

Best Friends

The single most important factor in a teen's decision to smoke is the behavior of his or her best friends of the same sex. A female teen whose best female friends all smoke is nearly six times as likely to smoke as our baseline teen with no smoking friends. The effect is even greater for boys than for girls: a male teen whose best friends all smoke is nearly eight times as likely to smoke. Indeed, the influence of same-sex peers is greater than the combined influence of having all best friends of the opposite sex smoke and having a steady boyfriend or girlfriend who smokes. Smoking by best friends of the opposite sex also matters, but it is less influential than the behavior of same-sex peers. A teen whose best friends of the opposite sex all smoke (but with no smoking best friends of the same sex) is only about 70 percent more likely to smoke. A teen with a steady boyfriend or girlfriend who is a smoker is just over twice as likely to smoke. Finally, a teen who says that most of his or her acquaintances (as opposed to best friends) smoke is about 80 percent more likely to smoke.

There are at least three possible explanations for the significance of peer behavior in determining teenage smoking decisions. First, teens may benefit socially from behavior that is similar to the behavior of their friends. Teens may perceive being part of a group as a benefit of smoking. Second, smoking is to some extent a social habit; it may simply be more pleasurable to smoke with others than to smoke alone. Finally, smoking among friends may effectively reduce the cost of smoking, because cigarettes are more readily available than they are to teens with no friends who smoke.

Perceived Benefits and Risks

The second set of factors influencing teenage smoking decisions is the individual teen's perceptions of the benefits and risks of smoking. It is these factors that provide some of the strongest evidence that teenage smoking decisions are rational. Rational teens would be more likely to smoke if they thought the benefits of smoking were greater, and less likely to smoke if they thought the risks were higher. Moreover, rational teens who dislike risk would be less likely to smoke. Actual teens behave in this fashion.

Teens were asked whether smoking helps when bored, whether it helps to relax, whether it helps deal with stress, and whether it helps to feel better in social situations. Teens who agree with all four measures are three times more likely to smoke than teens who do not. The only perceived benefit that is not individually important is the social benefit of smoking. Apparently, actual behavior of friends is a better measure of the social benefit of smoking than survey questions.

> *"There is . . . no reason to think that restrictions on advertising would have any influence on teenage smoking."*

Teens' opinions about the hazards of smoking also influence smoking decisions. Researchers, however, have seldom tried to determine teens' opinions of the actual magnitude of the risk of smoking. Surveys that try to do so have found that teens substantially overestimate the risk of smoking. More commonly, researchers ask teens whether an occasional cigarette is safe, and whether it is safe to smoke for a year or two. Although the "correct" answer to both questions is probably yes, two-thirds of teens think that even an occasional cigarette is harmful, and only 7 percent think that smoking for a year or two is safe.

Those who think it is safe to smoke an occasional cigarette are about 60 percent more likely to smoke. Teens who also think it is safe to smoke for a year or two are just over three times more likely to smoke. For teens who think that smoking is dangerous, attitudes about the ease of quitting are important. Teens who say they could quit any time they want to are almost twice as likely to smoke as teens who think they could not quit. Thus teens consider both risk and the difficulty of quitting in making decisions about smoking.

As one would expect, general attitudes toward risk are also important factors in predicting smoking behavior. Teens who report that they enjoy risky activities are 28 percent more likely to smoke than teens who are neutral about risk, and 63 percent more likely to smoke than teens who dislike risky activities.

Family Members

The third set of influences on teenage smoking decisions encompasses the smoking behavior of other family members. The most influential family members are older siblings. As with friends, same-sex siblings are more important than siblings of the opposite sex. An older, same-sex sibling who smokes more than doubles the likelihood of smoking, while opposite-sex siblings are less influential. Younger siblings who smoke have no significant influence on smoking decisions.

"Efforts to educate teens about the hazards of smoking have been quite successful."

The presence of adult smokers in the household also increases the likelihood that a teen will choose to smoke. Interestingly, however, the most influential adults are not parents. Instead, other adults—parents' partners or adult relatives—are more influential. Indeed, to the extent that teenage smoking reflects imitation of an adult role model, it appears that teens look to someone other than their parents as the model. If both parents are smokers, teens are slightly more likely to smoke, but the effect is not large enough to distinguish from simple chance. Indeed, the presence or absence of parents is more influential than their smoking behavior. Teens from households where one parent is not present are significantly more likely to smoke.

Advertising's Effect

Undoubtedly, the potential influence on teenage smoking that has most concerned policymakers is the role of advertising. Antismoking activists, congressmen, and the surgeon general have all argued for restrictions of one sort or another on the ability of the cigarette industry to tell consumers about its product, in the belief that the imagery accompanying such communications will lead vulnerable teens to take up smoking. From an economic perspective, however, the critical question is the kind of information conveyed by the cigarette advertisement. If the information is about brand-specific factors such as flavor (mild or strong, menthol or nonmenthol) or tar and nicotine content, there is no reason to expect any appreciable effect on teenage smoking decisions. The important factors motivating teenage smoking decisions are their perceptions of the benefits and risks of smoking, rather than the characteristics of particular brands. On the other hand, if advertising affects teens' perceptions of the benefits or risks of smoking, it could have some influence on smoking decisions.

The question is ultimately an empirical one that can only be answered by examining whether a teen's exposure to advertising messages influences his or her smoking decisions.

A 1990 survey of some 5,000 California teens commissioned by the State Department of Health makes possible just such an analysis. Because cigarette advertising varied in different California cities, and because it changed over time, there was substantial variation in the amount of cigarette advertising that individual teens might have seen. Indeed, the teens who were most exposed to advertising could have seen almost 2.5 times as much as the teens who were least exposed. If advertising influences teen decisions to smoke, teens in cities with more advertising or teens who were interviewed at times when advertising intensity was higher should have been more likely to be smokers.

In fact, they were not. Adding total cigarette advertising expenditures to the factors discussed above—peer behavior, perceptions of the risks and benefits of smoking, family influences—adds nothing to our ability to predict whether individual teens choose to smoke or not to smoke. Teens exposed to the most advertising are just as unlikely to smoke as teens exposed to the least advertising, once their other influences are taken into account.

Marlboro and Camel

Of course, different cigarette brands have different appeal to teens and adults. In California in 1990, the dominant brands among teens were Marlboro, with 63 percent of the teenage market, and Camel, with 22 percent. (Nationally, in 1989 Marlboro had 68 percent of the underage market, while Camel had 8 percent.) Perhaps it is only the advertising for these brands that influences teens' decisions about whether to smoke.

Again, however, there is no evidence of any such relationship. Teens who are most exposed to the advertising of either brand are no more likely to smoke than those who are least exposed. Once other factors that influence smoking decisions are considered, there is no detectable effect of the amount of advertising expenditures by the leading brands among teens.

In short, regardless of the measures of advertising or the definitions of smoking employed, any influence of advertising is not detectable. Whether smoking is defined as daily smoking,

> *"There is no discernible influence of cigarette advertising on decisions about smoking."*

smoking in the previous 30 days, or ever having smoked a single cigarette, the advertising expenditures of the industry or the inherent qualities of leading teenage brands have no influence on teens' decisions. Whether advertising expenditures are measured over the previous three months or the previous three years, there is no detectable influence. Whether measures of the perceived benefits of smoking that might be attributable to advertising are included or excluded, advertising expenditures have no detectable effect. There is, in short, no reason to think that restrictions on advertising would have any influence on teenage smoking.

There is one policy alternative that has been shown to reduce teenage smoking. Although virtually every state prohibits sales of cigarettes to teens under a certain age (usually 18), these laws are often only weakly enforced. Studies of communities that have launched enforcement campaigns, however, have found significant declines in teenage smoking. But calls for stricter enforcement of local ordinances simply lack the political appeal and potential for publicity available from attacks on cigarette advertising, hence their relative scarcity.

Policymakers Have Little Control

Teenage smoking has been declining and continues to do so. Efforts to educate teens about the hazards of smoking have been quite successful, with virtually all teens recognizing that smoking poses risks. Rather than acknowledging this substantial progress, however, some argue for ever more draconian steps to control teenage smoking. While any teenage smoking is regrettable and should surely be discouraged, policymakers have little control over most factors influencing teen smoking. Despite its visibility, there is no discernible influence of cigarette advertising on decisions about smoking. Teens' decisions about smoking are fundamentally rational, determined by the balance between the perceived benefits and risks of smoking. Like other forms of youthful experimentation with adult behaviors, ranging from illegal drugs to sex and alcohol use, some teenage smoking will undoubtedly continue. So too will calls from activists of various stripes and the politicians who seek their support to "do something," regardless of whether it will actually work.

Government Measures to Reduce Teen Smoking Are Counterproductive

by Thomas Humber

About the author: *Thomas Humber is president and CEO of the National Smokers Alliance, an organization that opposes discrimination against smokers.*

In 1995, the National Smokers Alliance ran a series of national ads, the principal theme of which was "Defending smokers' rights protects everyone's." The ads had multiple purposes, including social experiment. They referred to the "extremism of the life-style police," and, judging by calls and mail we received from antismokers, extremism is too mild a term.

The callers were abusive, obscene, and, on occasion, threatening. Some were dismaying in their ignorance. Most were chilling in their arrogant certitude and elitism. One citizen of our free society scrawled "Kill all smokers" and similar comments across the ads in blood red ink and sent them to us, one by one, as they appeared.

The Antismoking Brigade

"Kill" is, of course, language of the streets, of those who live with pent-up hostility in extremis, to whom solutions of finality seem perfectly appropriate for those they dislike. The language of government is regulation.

Bill Clinton, guided by political advisers with desperate fingers in the whirling political wind, has determined that he, too, must officially join the antismoking brigade by giving the Food and Drug Administration (FDA) jurisdiction to regulate tobacco products. The stated purpose is to reduce teenage smoking.

That the ultimate goal is the prohibition of a legal product is steadfastly denied. The denials are believed by no grown-up who can function without a guardian. Some FDA watchers question the wisdom of placing *any* product under the control of a commissioner who, as one of his first official acts, ordered U.S. marshals

Thomas Humber, "Teenage Smoking: Kids Can Think for Themselves." This article appeared in the December 1995 issue and is reprinted with permission from the *World & I*, a publication of The Washington Times Corporation, copyright © 1995.

to seize and destroy 12,000 gallons of orange juice because the label—which used the word *fresh* when the product was made from concentrate—was "misleading." Most governments can only dream of the plenty that would allow such excessive behavior.

Most adult Americans—including smokers—believe that minors should not smoke, just as they believe that minors should not consume alcohol, use illicit drugs, or carry their firearms to school. Had the imposition of adult beliefs ever produced any but the opposite of the intended effect on the behavior of minors, rock and roll would not have lasted long enough to have a Hall of Fame.

> *"Ask yourself if you honestly believe that . . . restrictions on cigarette advertising . . . will curtail teenage smoking."*

Set aside, for one moment, the rhetoric of the political panderers and ask yourself if you honestly believe that the elimination of cigarette vending machines, decals on racing cars, and restrictions on cigarette advertising—the proposed FDA solutions—will curtail teenage smoking.

Can Extra Laws Save Us?

Apply, for one moment, the common sense logic that government and those who would save us from ourselves have cynically abandoned. The incidence of smoking among teenagers had been steadily declining for some years. Over the same period, the advertising, promotion, and distribution activities of the cigarette manufacturers remained relatively static, yet the incidence of smoking among teenagers recently trended upward. What changed?

The antismoking rhetoric. It exploded in an organized, orchestrated effort, from the bully pulpit of politics, from overflowing coffers of cigarette tax money earmarked for antismoking "education." Cause and effect? Perhaps not, but the details fit recognizable patterns and the psychology of youth rebellion.

Does it occur to no one in the federal government that, just perhaps, the almost-forgotten concept and application of parental guidance might be more useful than yet another government program with regard to teenage smoking and a number of other issues as well?

Because the efforts proposed by the FDA will not work, the FDA will obviously be "forced" to enact even more draconian measures, all the while proclaiming that prohibition is nowhere in the plan, until it arrives.

Perspective

As with many other issues that distance politicians from those who elected them, it is time for some perspective.

To smoke is to engage in a risky personal life-style choice. Fifty million adult smokers do it. I am one of those, and I smoke with full understanding of the risks—and the benefits—of that choice. While I owe explanation or apology to no one, I do owe nonsmokers courtesy and consideration if the proximity of my smoking bothers them. I also owe my fellow citizens respect for their personal life-style choices, whether or not I agree with them.

This country was born of rebellion against authoritarianism and founded upon the principles of freedom and tolerance. Yet, despite our best efforts, tolerance for individual differences has been difficult to achieve and even more so to maintain. We are, after all, human and not nearly so civilized as we pretend.

In an increasingly fractured society, smokers are being cast as the new pariahs. Why that is true is complicated. It involves a recent and distinctly generational aversion to any risk, real or perceived. It also involves our growing culture of confrontation, elements of mass psychology, the power of suggestion, the shortage of politically correct targets, the inability of government to deal with other social concerns, and even guaranteed media coverage for politicians and activists who attack smoking.

A Reversal in Civil Liberties

The attack on smoking has produced a frightening reversal in the progress of civil liberties. For decades, business owners and employers have been told they could discriminate against no one. Now they are increasingly told they *must* discriminate against smokers, regardless of the effect on their businesses.

In California, a law that began taking effect in January 1995 and mandates the exclusion of smoking from business establishments statewide already has taken a toll on small business. Restaurants, coffeehouses, billiard parlors, bowling alleys, and bingo facilities are losing customers and income, for the establishments and for their employees. Some will fail, through no fault of their own, after years of building their clientele, smoking and nonsmoking. Yet those who would control all aspects of our lives will have moved on to their next cause, proud they have protected their space, even though that space may be closed to all.

In New York City, where similar legislation was implemented in April 1995, 70 percent of restaurant owners responding to a September 1995 survey reported losses averaging approximately 16 percent, with more than 40 percent of that group reporting forced layoffs.

> *"The incidence of smoking among teenagers had been steadily declining for some years."*

"Your freedom ends where our noses begin" is the unremitting response of the antismoking crusaders, seeking, not unsuccessfully, to push the hot buttons of victimization. This attitude, coupled with the EPA's January 1993 report on "environmental tobacco smoke," has fueled the intensity of today's debate.

Nothing I can say on the subject will change the public's perception of its dangers. Most scientists with the credentials, objectivity, and credibility to set the record straight have no desire to detour from more serious pursuits to enter this political muck.

Instructive Voices

It is instructive, however, to hear some voices.

Writing in *Toxicologic Pathology*, Dr. Alvan Feinstein, professor of medicine and epidemiology at Yale University School of Medicine, quoted an "authoritative leader in the world of public health epidemiology" (charitably unnamed): "Yes, it's rotten science, but it's in a worthy cause. It will help us get rid of cigarettes and become a smoke-free society."

After one of the few independent and substantial analyses of the EPA report, Jane Gravelle, senior specialist in economic policy of the Congressional Research Service, testified before a congressional committee that "our evaluation was that the statistical evidence does not appear to support a conclusion that there were substantial health effects of passive smoking."

Dr. Morton Lippmann, who chaired the EPA Science Advisory Board committee that reviewed the EPA study, was asked at a news conference to put the risk in perspective. His response was that the possibility of cancer from second-hand smoke is "a small added risk, probably much less than you took to get here through Washington traffic."

"To me, it's frightening that they could make such a case out of such a small risk factor when you've got so many variables," says Dr. James Engstrom, a professor of epidemiology at UCLA.

Speaking Against the Mob

There are others, but they speak against the mob. Whatever one's viewpoint, those voices suggest that something is wrong; all is not as it appears.

The majority of smokers understand that the accommodation we seek is a two-way street. The majority of smokers are asking only the fairness and tolerance that are required in any nation that respects individual differences. The majority of smokers are nonconfrontational, but each day's affront provokes a rising level of bitterness and anger, as well as increasing activism and commitment to the preservation of their individual choice.

Smokers are now a minority, in numbers and in treatment. But 50 million smokers are a powerful political and economic force. Fewer than 50 million people voted for the current president of the United States. The money of 50 million people is the profit margin of America.

Do smokers have rights? That is a political question, and the answer for smokers, as it has been for others, is, not if we do not fight for them. We agreed to be governed; we did not agree to be controlled.

Chapter 5

Should Government Regulation of Smoking Be Increased?

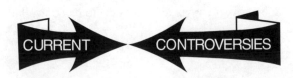

Government Regulation of Smoking: An Overview

by Hank Cox

About the author: *Hank Cox is a contributor to* Insight on the News, *a weekly newsmagazine, and works for the Washington, D.C., Chamber of Commerce.*

In February 1995, Cindy Gilmer flew from Starkville, Miss., to the nation's capital to testify before the Occupational Safety and Health Administration. The experience, she said later, was a "real eye-opener."

Gilmer owns and operates a billiards hall, the sort of establishment in which smoking is de rigueur. OSHA wants to outlaw smoking in the workplace, including restaurants and pool rooms. "You can't just throw a blanket over business and treat us all the same," says Gilmer. "A lot of us do not need, and certainly cannot afford, to spend $10,000 on a separate smoking room. It just doesn't make any sense."

The Antismoking Drive

Even as the Clinton administration championed a hefty 75-cents-per-pack tax increase on cigarettes to fund health care reform, Congress was publicly chastising tobacco executives. In April 1994, Rep. Henry Waxman, a Democrat from California and then-chairman of the Energy and Commerce subcommittee on health and the environment, seemed to revel in the role of righteous avenger as he grilled the heads of the six leading tobacco companies. The antismoking drive had kicked into overdrive.

In February 1994, for example, McDonald's Corp. banned smoking in all of its 11,000 restaurants, prompting other restaurant chains to follow suit. Within days, the Department of Defense imposed a worldwide ban on smoking at military bases. The same month, the Food and Drug Administration began to consider classifying nicotine as a regulated drug.

The antismoking lobby and the tobacco industry were headed for a major legislative showdown when the November election ushered in a conservative landslide, ceding control of key House committees to Republicans, who are less interested in regulating behavior by legislative fiat. "The biggest setback was an end to the investigation," an aide to Waxman said. "The tobacco industry had agreed to surrender all internal documents relating to health effects. Now we'll never see them."

State and Local Restrictions

The shift in tobacco's fortunes in Congress was not reflected on state and local levels, however. Since 1985, the number of local governments restricting smoking has increased from 45 to more than 600. Even anarchic New York City has adopted a comprehensive smoking ordinance, for the first time extending smoking restrictions to outdoor areas such as parks and stadiums. "This is where the rest of the world is going," explained Mayor Rudolph Giuliani.

Meanwhile, California withstood an assault on its antismoking law. Proposition 188, heavily backed by the tobacco industry during the November 1994 election, would have overturned not only the state measure but local antismoking ordinances as well. "Even though Philip Morris outspent the opposition 20-to-1," says Cathy Leonard, who works for the State Assembly's Committee on Labor and Employment, "Proposition 188 got less than 29 percent of the vote."

Maryland has instituted one of the most comprehensive antismoking ordinances in the nation. State health officials had proposed a ban on smoking not only in office buildings, but also in bars, restaurants and convention centers, although Democratic Gov. Parris Glendening has led a compromise effort to allow smoking in bars. At any rate, the Maryland antismoking measure will be the first instituted not by legislators

> *"The antismoking lobby and the tobacco industry were headed for a major legislative showdown."*

or voters, but by bureaucrats. "Both parties support restrictions on smoking," says Peter Fisher of the Coalition on Smoking or Health, a Washington organization that educates policymakers on tobacco-control topics. "It is a bipartisan issue."

Indeed, cigarette manufacturers, tobacco farmers and smokers are losing the war as well as the battles over smoking. According to the Centers for Disease Control and Prevention, the number of American adults who smoke has decreased by almost half during the last 30 years, from a little more than 42 percent of the population in 1965 to about 25 percent in 1995. Nevertheless, while health officials hope to eradicate smoking altogether, they face formidable financial reality.

Tobacco Money

Tobacco is a major agricultural crop in the United States, especially in the Southeast, with total farm sales of $2.8 billion in 1993. That year, the major tobacco companies grossed $50 billion from domestic sales and another $5.7 billion in foreign sales, reporting more than $5 billion in net profits. Perhaps more importantly, excise taxes collected on tobacco products, mainly cigarettes, exceed $13 billion annually, or more than four times the total value of tobacco products raised on the farm. That money supports many government programs.

According to a 1992 study by Price Waterhouse, the tobacco industry accounts for more than 680,000 jobs.

In addition, members of Congress, despite their public stands on smoking, are not adverse to tobacco money. According to *Common Cause* magazine, 73 percent of senators accepted campaign contributions from tobacco companies between 1989 and 1994; 66 percent of congressmen took tobacco money in the 1994 House election. Critics claim this "tainted" money extracts a far bigger price on society. According to the Department of Health and Human Services, tobacco-related illness costs society $50 billion annually.

> *"The number of American adults who smoke has decreased by almost half during the last 30 years."*

Risks and Costs

While few people deny the hazards of smoking, some researchers claim that the risks are exaggerated and social costs inflated. A 1991 study by the Rand Corp. put the net external cost of cigarette smoking at 33 cents per pack; since existing federal, state and local taxes on cigarettes total more than 50 cents per pack, smokers more than pay their own way.

The impact of tobacco on the nation's economy becomes even more smoky when Social Security and other pension programs are factored in. John Shoven, an economist at Stanford University, estimates that the 26 billion packs of cigarettes smoked in 1989 shortened smokers' lives by 3 million years, and that their premature deaths saved $20,000 per smoker in Social Security benefits alone. The Congressional Research Service, in a report issued March 8, 1994, observed that "smokers' early deaths leave their Social Security and pension contributions unused and available to reduce future financing demands on nonsmokers."

More controversial still is the issue of secondary smoke. The Environmental Protection Agency in 1993 claimed secondary smoke was responsible for up to 3,000 cases of lung cancer annually. But the EPA report has been challenged by a diverse array of credible scientists. EPA performed no original research but relied instead on a survey of 30 other studies, of which only six discerned a statistically significant (but small) effect of secondary smoke on nonsmokers. Of the remaining 24 studies, six actually showed a reduced incidence of illness among those exposed to secondary smoke.

Price Supports

While the Clinton administration and major federal agencies target tobacco for strict regulation, other branches of the national government continue their long-established tradition of supporting prices and allotting production quotas. The Tobacco Institute insists tobacco is not subsidized; strictly speaking, it isn't. But the Rube Goldberg scheme that controls tobacco production, a holdover from the New Deal of the 1930s, is wildly out of step with the free-market agenda now dominant in Congress.

Only people who own "quotas" can legally grow and sell tobacco, and quotas are passed along from generation to generation. A large number of people who inherited tobacco quotas do not actually grow any crop. Currently, there are 380,000 quota holders but only 100,000 tobacco farmers—those farmers pay the quota holders a fee for use.

Tobacco farmers are guaranteed minimum prices through price supports in exchange for limiting production. Most of these subsidy costs are paid by producers and purchasers through market assessments. (Administrative costs of about $15 million a year are borne by taxpayers.) The sum effect: The price of tobacco stays higher than it would in a free market, while excessive supplies of the crop accumulate in warehouses.

Imports and Exports

As foreign nations stepped up competition and made it more difficult for the United States to maintain artificially inflated price levels, the domestic tobacco industry lobbied Congress to limit imports of foreign tobacco. Since 1993, any U.S. cigarette maker who uses more than 25 percent of foreign tobacco must pay a penalty. Foreign producers naturally complain that price supports violate the General Agreement on Tariffs and Trade, created specifically to discourage arbitrary barriers to imports and exports. Industry experts worry that when Congress is forced to address this problem, it simply will eliminate price supports.

But federal bureaucracies promote and defend tobacco exports overseas. In recent years, the U.S. trade representative has helped gain access for U.S. tobacco exports to Japan, Taiwan, Thailand and South Korea. China is the biggest plum of all, offering a market of 300 million smokers. In 1992, the United States persuaded China to begin opening its market to cigarettes and several other products by threatening to impose 300 percent tariffs on almost $4 billion worth of Chinese imports.

"While few people deny the hazards of smoking, some researchers claim that the risks are exaggerated and social costs inflated."

The Clinton administration has set up an interagency task force to review policy on tobacco exports. According to spokesman Chris Marcich, the goal is to ensure that health concerns raised by foreign nations about U.S. cigarettes are not a ruse to protect their domestic brands from U.S. competition. "We expect our trading partners to live up to their agreements," Marcich says. "Just as we expect foreign cigarette makers selling their product here to apply warning labels, we will honor their health-related requirements and restrictions."

Lawsuits

Perhaps the greatest threat to the tobacco industry emanates not from Congress, state and local governments or even foreign competitors, but from courts of law. During the last four decades, the tobacco industry has attracted more than 300 lawsuits attempting to establish liability for smoking-related illnesses, thus far without success. But 1994 brought an avalanche of litigation, possibly stimulated by stepped-up antismoking activity elsewhere, and several states have joined the fray.

Minnesota, along with Blue Cross/Blue Shield of Minnesota and the law firm of Robins, Kaplan, Miller & Ciresi, is suing the Big Six tobacco companies. The lawsuit differs from others, however; the team is focusing not on the hazardous products sold by tobacco companies, but on their conduct in promoting their products.

Mississippi, West Virginia and Florida also have joined in the effort to force tobacco companies to help pay the medical costs of patients with tobacco-related illnesses. "Florida's taxpayers consistently have to make withdrawals from their wallets to pay for the carnage," says Florida Gov. Lawton Chiles.

Most ambitious yet: A federal judge in New Orleans cleared the way for a gigantic, nationwide class-action suit by a consortium of 60 law firms on behalf of 100 million smokers and former smokers.

According to Michael Pertschuk, codirector of the Advocacy Institute in Washington, tobacco companies spend more than $600 million on legal fees annually, and the figure is rising. Increasingly, the industry is taking the offensive. Philip Morris filed a $10 billion suit in 1994 against ABC News after a network program accused the company of adding nicotine to its product to keep smokers addicted. In the summer of 1994, several tobacco companies sued the EPA over its report about secondary tobacco smoke.

One further concern has been raised by the new chairman of the House Energy and Commerce subcommittee on health and the environment. "The antismoking people say they don't really want a ban," Rep. Thomas J. Bliley, a Republican from Virginia, said. "But that would be the logical result of what they are doing. If federal agencies should ban smoking, and the

> *"Federal bureaucracies promote and defend tobacco exports overseas."*

lawyers put the tobacco companies out of business, the result will be a thriving black market on top of the existing black market for illegal drugs. What will be the impact of that on this country? They don't think about that."

151

Smoking Should Be Strictly Regulated

by Hobart Rowen

About the author: *Hobart Rowen is a syndicated columnist whose articles often appear in* Liberal Opinion Week, *a newspaper of liberal political opinion.*

Tobacco may have caused more than 400,000 premature American deaths in 1993, but never underrate the power of the tobacco lobby. With Dan Rostenkowski now on the sidelines, a House Ways and Means subcommittee lowered a proposed tax on cigarettes to a meaningless 60 cents per pack over six years.

Sixty cents is less than half of the Rosty-endorsed subcommittee proposal of a $1.25 tax, and below the 75 cents in the Clinton health plan—both watered way down from the $2 a pack first considered by the White House.

That would not only cut the revenue for financing health care reform, but would barely, if at all, be reflected in retail cigarette prices. Thus, it would do little to discourage smoking or the sale of cigarettes. That's why cigarette stock prices on the New York Stock Exchange rose in response to the news.

A Groundswell of Opposition

But the last word has not been heard on this subject. Despite the setback in the Ways and Means subcommittee, I think the tobacco interests are at last meeting a groundswell of important opposition. A United States District Court squelched the attempt by one company to intimidate or silence two Congressional critics, Reps. Ron Wyden (D. Ore.) and Henry Waxman (D. Calif.).

Another highly significant development: according to Congressional sources, the Clinton Administration has decided . . . it won't pursue "Section 301" punitive trade actions against our trading partners at the behest of American companies seeking further penetration of overseas tobacco markets.

"I think the American companies are trying to muddle the picture here, to stall action for a few years until they can extend their foothold in the Asian market, and hook and addict millions of Chinese and other children," Wyden told me.

Smoking Must Be Restricted

I sense a growing feeling in America that the availability of cigarettes for minors must be drastically limited. Kids— even grade-schoolers—have easy access to cigarettes through vending machines. The existing ban on sale of cigarettes to minors under 18 is a joke.

Smoking and the production of cigarettes can be made subject to greater government regulation. Already, smoking has been banned on U.S. military bases, airlines, passenger trains, and by many private companies in their workplaces. Smoking need not be banned outright. But those who choose to risk the hazards of cigarettes should have to do so in controlled situations where the air they pollute does not directly affect non-smokers.

A few states have banned most workplace smoking, and Florida has launched an innovative attack that seeks to recover from tobacco companies the public costs of dealing with disease traceable to cigarette smoking. In some states, as happened recently in Wisconsin, the lobby has been able to defeat modest attempts to curb smoking in public places and shopping malls.

Is there a negative side to regulation of smoking? As former president Jimmy Carter has said, one must feel compassion for the "plight of the tobacco farmer," who has been encouraged by the cigarette-makers to produce ever larger quantities for domestic consumption and for export.

But as Carter noted, change in the tobacco economy of the South is already occurring. Many farmers have seen that diversification is necessary in their own self-interest.

Congressmen Wyden and Waxman have performed a public service by exposing the possibility that various companies suppressed data on smoking addiction for as much as 30 years. They have joined with more than 40 other colleagues in an effort to bring the tobacco industry under the general control of the Food and Drug Administration.

> *"Smoking . . . can be made subject to greater government regulation."*

In a separate bill, Waxman would be more specific. Among his many good ideas: A ban on industry sponsorship of sporting events, such as tennis tournaments, unless the companies pass out information on the effects of smoking on health at such events. He would also make illegal the distribution of free cigarette samples.

A License to Smoke

Another provocative idea—advanced by 45-year-old anti-tobacco crusader Patrick Reynolds—whose inheritance came from the producers of Camel cigarettes, the R.J. Reynolds tobacco company—is to raise the age for purchasing cigarettes to 21, not 18, and require merchants to have a license to sell cigarettes, just as they do for booze.

I can hear the tobacco lobbyists chanting, "What, you tell a kid that he can be drafted into the army at 18, but can't buy cigarettes until he's 21?" The answer is "Yes!" A determined nation can make that stick. In an interview in the *Los Angeles Times*, Reynolds cited statistics showing that 60 per cent of smokers start by the age of 14, and 90 per cent by the age of 19: "If we can keep cigarettes away from kids until they're 21, we would go a long way toward eliminating the problem."

The fight against the tobacco industry will be uphill all the way. It is rich and powerful. But the battle can be won. Who would have bet a couple of years ago that the airlines would have the guts to ban smoking on all flights, or that newspapers would send their smokers out of the newsrooms and into the streets?

The FDA Should Regulate the Tobacco Industry

by Scott D. Ballin

About the author: *Scott D. Ballin is chairman of the Coalition on Smoking OR Health, a group that works to decrease smoking through education and government regulation.*

David Kessler, the United States Food and Drug Administration commissioner, is attempting to bring the tobacco industry under his agency's control. The president and Congress should firmly and publicly back Dr. Kessler as he seeks to regulate tobacco companies.

Congress and the Tobacco Industry

The tobacco industry occupies a special place among Washington's special interests. One need not look further than the Senate gutting of a proposed tobacco tax that would have helped finance health-care reform. Two Senate committees—Labor and Human Resources and Finance—approved health-care language that included $1.50- and $1-per-pack tobacco taxes, respectively. The members of those committees knew that the majority of Americans were willing to accept a significant tobacco-tax increase, even up to $2 per pack. What happened? When Sen. George Mitchell (D) of Maine announced his bill, the tobacco tax had wilted to 45 cents per pack, phased in over five years. It seems that the new Senate math is being taught by the tobacco lobby.

The tobacco industry has always had its way with Congress. Just ask the Tobacco Institute, the Washington-based lobbying arm for the tobacco industry. On numerous occasions, it has taken to publicly proclaiming satisfaction with the legislative process on Capitol Hill. Kessler knows this lesson all too well. By publicly turning up the heat on tobacco regulation, he's thrown a sabot into the tobacco industry's wheel of fortune. It's one thing for the tobacco industry to lobby Congress, where the money spigot is always open and running. Muscling aside a determined FDA commissioner may be another story.

Scott D. Ballin, "Put Tobacco Regulation Under the FDA," *Christian Science Monitor*, October 13, 1994. Reprinted with permission.

Slanted Tobacco Survey

Clearly Kessler believes tobacco is an enormous public health problem, as does the world's health community. The potential for preventing a generation of young people from becoming hooked on tobacco and becoming statistics in the next round of smoking-related deaths appears to be his motivation to bring tobacco under FDA regulation. The tobacco industry has responded with attempts to color Kessler a prohibitionist. It even includes that language in its national survey questions to ensure that it can falsely portray a public dissatisfaction with regulating tobacco.

For example, a Roper Starch telephone survey commissioned by R.J. Reynolds asks the question: "Do you think the federal government should regulate the purchase, use, and production of tobacco products if such regulations would likely result in the prohibition of cigarettes or smoking . . . ?" A Gallup survey commissioned by our coalition asked a different question and found that 68 percent of Americans—both smokers and nonsmokers—believe that tobacco products should be regulated by the FDA in a manner similar to how drugs are regulated.

What approach is Kessler likely to take to regulate tobacco? In a letter sent to our coalition, Kessler said he was asking Congress for "guidance" on the issue. So far, nothing concrete has emerged from Capitol Hill. The most logical step for Congress to take would be to . . . give the FDA the same clear-cut authority to regulate tobacco it currently has for foods, drugs, and cosmetics. . . .

> *"The president and Congress should firmly and publicly back Dr. Kessler as he seeks to regulate tobacco companies."*

But Kessler can propose regulations for tobacco without congressional action. He appears to be interested in ratcheting down nicotine levels in cigarettes to below an addictive threshold, which is yet to be agreed upon by the scientific community. That action could keep cigarettes from a drug classification, but they would still be a dangerous product.

For the past decade, the Coalition on Smoking OR Health has advocated FDA regulation of tobacco products as one of the most effective and reasonable approaches to tobacco control. At a minimum, FDA regulation of tobacco should encompass the following:

Manufacturing: Require the tobacco industry to disclose to the public the levels of nicotine, tar, chemical additives, and all other potentially harmful substances in tobacco products.

Sales: Require the enforcement of laws so that tobacco products are not sold to anyone under the age of 21.

Labeling: Require all tobacco products to carry warnings on addiction, chemical additives, and other information critical to public health. The FDA should prohibit use of misleading claims in both the labeling and advertising of to-bacco products.

Advertising: Ban all tobacco advertising targeted at children. The FDA should ban or restrict deceptive or misleading images for all tobacco advertising as is done for other products.

Promotion: Ban free or discounted giveaways of tobacco products. The FDA should eliminate the sponsorship of any event, such as a sports or arts event, that uses the brand name of a tobacco product.

Don't Ban, but Regulate

The public-health community must continue to help smokers who want to quit, and do everything it can to prevent children and teenagers from starting to smoke. Our health organizations have worked with millions of smokers who want to quit. We know how difficult it can be. A ban will not work. But we are in the midst of a tobacco epidemic. Smoking is expected to kill 419,000 Americans each year. It adds $30 billion annually in direct medical costs to our national health-care bill. The suffering it causes individuals and families is immeasurable.

Tobacco regulation is a straightforward and admirable public-health goal. It is perfectly in line with the FDA's responsibility and the government's role in public-health and safety issues. Congress has a choice: Give in once more to tobacco special interests or work with Kessler. For his part, President Clinton can show that he means it when he inveighs against special-interest politics. He should stand behind his FDA commissioner while he stands up to the tobacco industry.

Tobacco Taxes Should Be Increased

by Jimmy Carter

About the author: *Jimmy Carter was president of the United States from 1976 to 1980. Prior to his term in the White House, he served as governor of Georgia. He is currently involved in Habitat for Humanity, an organization that helps low-income people build their own homes.*

As our president searches for ways to improve health care and reduce budget deficits, he should seriously consider a major increase in federal tobacco taxes. He could save hundreds of thousands of lives and simultaneously raise tens of billions of dollars for health care reform or deficit reduction.

Suffering and Loss

I know the incalculable toll of suffering and human loss caused by tobacco use. My father, my mother, both sisters, and my brother died of cancer. Every one of them smoked cigarettes. Each year nearly one-half million Americans die from direct and passive smoking.

The U.S. Centers for Disease Control and Prevention estimates that direct use of tobacco kills more than 8,300 Americans each week. This is roughly double the total of all deaths caused by alcohol, car accidents, AIDS, suicide, homicide, fires, crack cocaine, and heroin. In addition, the Environmental Protection Agency (EPA) has classified environmental tobacco smoke as a known human carcinogen that causes lung cancer and death among non-smokers. The EPA also found that exposure to environmental tobacco smoke is particularly dangerous for children and babies.

The single most effective way to reduce tobacco use and nicotine addiction, especially among children, is to increase substantially the price of tobacco products. The country's leading health organizations, including the American Cancer Society, American Lung Association, American Heart Association, and American Medical Association, are urging President Clinton and Congress to

Jimmy Carter, "Proposed Tobacco Tax Would Raise Money and Save Lives," *Carter Center of Emory University News*, Spring 1993. Reprinted by permission of the American Cancer Society, Inc.

raise the cigarette excise tax $2 a pack.

Our children are the most important reason for a major tobacco tax increase. We know that 90 percent of all smokers begin as teenagers, who are more sensitive to higher prices than adults. We can deter millions of young people from ever starting to smoke, saving hundreds of thousands of them from addiction and premature death. Health groups estimate that a $2-a-pack tax increase would reduce smoking rates enough to save nearly 2 million lives—more than the total lives lost in all U.S. wars combined.

> *"The single most effective way to reduce tobacco use . . . is to increase . . . the price of tobacco products."*

This proposal would raise more than $30 billion a year in new revenue that could be put to good use funding health care reform, childhood immunization efforts, and other high priorities. In this way, tobacco could begin to pay its fair share of the tremendous costs it imposes on our society, including the estimated half-trillion dollars in health care costs for current smokers.

It is a bitter irony that cigarette taxes were twice as high in real terms in the 1950s, before we knew the lethal and addictive nature of this product, than they are today. While a $2-a-pack tax increase may sound high, it would only begin to bring U.S. tobacco tax rates into line with other industrialized nations. Canada, for example, has seen a 40 percent decline in smoking since it raised its tobacco taxes from rates comparable to the United States to more than $3 a pack. While teenage smoking rates in the United States have remained persistently high, teen smoking in Canada has fallen by two-thirds since taxes began rising in the early 1980s.

A Tax Would Help the Poor

Tobacco manufacturers will argue that tobacco taxes disproportionately affect the poor. Yet, it is the industry's own marketing activities that have the most regressive impact, targeting the youngest, poorest, and least educated for addiction—those groups least able to afford the added health care costs. Economists expect higher tobacco taxes to have a highly positive economic impact on low-income communities when long-term health benefits are considered. These benefits would be even greater if tobacco tax revenues are used to fund programs that serve the poor.

In addition to health and economic benefits, tobacco taxes are the most popular revenue-raising option. This has been confirmed by national polls and by voters themselves in statewide referenda to raise tobacco taxes.

We have before us a measure that could save 2 million American lives and raise $30 billion in annual revenues. Especially for our children, I urge President Clinton and the Congress to take this historic opportunity and boost the tobacco tax.

Increased Regulation of Smoking Would Strengthen the Economy

by Kenneth E. Warner and George A. Fulton

About the authors: *Kenneth E. Warner is a professor of public health policy and administration at the University of Michigan in Ann Arbor. George A. Fulton is a research scientist in the Department of Economics and Institute of Labor and Industrial Relations at the University of Michigan.*

Since the late 1970s, the tobacco industry has relied increasingly on an economic argument as a public relations defense against proposed tobacco-control measures. The industry has attempted to convince legislators, journalists, and the general public that, regardless of its effects on physical health, tobacco plays a critical role in their communities' economic health, generating employment and contributing vital revenues to government coffers. The industry contends that regulatory measures that reduce smoking and hence cigarette sales, such as clean indoor air laws, will increase unemployment and government deficits. (In the case of one policy measure of contemporary interest, cigarette excise taxation, the industry's argument relates only to employment, since higher taxes clearly will increase tax revenues.)

To develop its economic argument, the industry has commissioned consultants to estimate the economic contribution of tobacco to the nation as a whole and to the individual states, including the employment generated by production, distribution, and sale of tobacco products; compensation associated with the employment; and government revenues from taxes on the sale of tobacco products and on associated employment and business income. Findings from these studies are transmitted to legislators, journalists, and other interested parties when legislative proposals threaten cigarette sales, particularly in nontobacco states. Economic dependence on tobacco is a less obvious concern in the nontobacco states than in the half dozen southeastern tobacco states.

From Kenneth E. Warner and George A. Fulton, "The Economic Implications of Tobacco Product Sales in a Nontobacco State," *JAMA*, vol. 271, no. 10, p. 771-76, March 9, 1994. Copyright 1994, American Medical Association. Reprinted with permission.

Reallocated Spending

The industry's estimates greatly exaggerate tobacco's economic importance. Implicitly, they treat the resources devoted to tobacco product production and distribution as disappearing if sales decline or cease altogether. However, the amount of economic activity associated with tobacco product sales would not disappear if consumers decreased or even ceased their spending on tobacco products. Rather, it would be redistributed as consumers used the same money to purchase alternative goods and services. Just like spending on tobacco, this alternative spending would generate employment and tax revenues associated with the production, distribution, and sale of purchased goods and services.

In most or possibly all nontobacco states, the reallocated spending might be expected to produce more employment than does tobacco. A sizable proportion of the dollars consumers spend on tobacco products are "exported" to the tobacco states—half in the case of our state, Michigan. If reallocated, a larger proportion of the spending might be on goods and services indigenous to the nontobacco state. As a consequence, a higher percentage of the dollars would be recycled within the state's economy, thereby generating greater local economic activity than did the expenditures on tobacco.

To evaluate the net effect of this reallocation in a nontobacco state, we employed a state-of-the-art macroeconomic model to simulate the consequences of consumers' reducing their tobacco expenditures in Michigan, with the same level of spending redistributed to other goods and services according to consumers' normal spending patterns. We considered two cases: the complete and instantaneous cessation of tobacco expenditures and an acceleration in the current rate of decline in tobacco consumption in Michigan. . . .

Tobacco Sales, Employment, and Taxes

We estimated that, in 1992, tobacco product sales in Michigan generated 7843 "direct employment" jobs (those directly related to the distribution and sale of tobacco products within the state), concentrated heavily (over 90%) in the retail and wholesale trade sectors. In addition to direct employment, we estimated that tobacco spending was responsible for 11,284 spin-off jobs in the state: 2159 "indirect" jobs (generated by increased purchases from Michigan suppliers) and 9125 "induced" jobs (resulting from spending by people who receive income due to tobacco product sales); the induced employment includes 5333 government jobs. Thus, when we combined direct, indirect, and induced employment, tobacco product sales in Michigan were associated with a total of 19,127 jobs in the state in 1992, or just under 0.5% of total state employment.

"The tobacco industry has relied increasingly on an economic argument as a public relations defense."

According to official state figures, cigarette sales generated $245 million in excise tax revenues in Michigan in calendar year 1992, approximately $60 million in general sales taxes, and much smaller amounts in related personal and business income taxes.

Impact on Employment

Table 1 presents our estimates of the gross and net impacts on employment of completely eliminating tobacco product sales in Michigan for selected years from 1992 through 2005 (columns 1 through 3) and the redistribution of jobs by sector in a Michigan economy with no tobacco product sales (columns 4 through 7). The first column indicates the gross number of tobacco-related jobs that would have been lost in the Michigan economy if tobacco expenditures had ceased completely and instantly in 1992. The figure for 1992 is thus the gross employment contribution in Michigan of in-state tobacco sales, reported in the preceding section. After accounting for a continuation of the expected "normal" decline in tobacco expenditures, the gross number of tobacco-related jobs that would be lost due to cessation of tobacco expenditures would fall gradually to just over 14,000 by the year 2005.

Column 2 of Table 1 shows our estimates of the gross employment that would replace that generated by tobacco sales, were such sales ended and the equivalent amount of money redirected to consumption expenditures on other goods and services. Column 3 then presents the sum of the gross employment impacts (with and without tobacco), yielding the net change in employment in Michigan that would result from the elimination of spending on tobacco products: 5608 more jobs in 1992 without tobacco, falling to 1478 more jobs in the year 2005 (again, after accounting for the expected continuation of the "normal" decline in tobacco expenditures). Columns 4 through 7 show the distribution of these additional jobs: small losses in employment in the sectors most dependent on tobacco product sales—retail trade, wholesale trade, and state and local government (reflecting lost cigarette excise tax revenues)—and, as shown in column 7,

Table 1.—Gross and Net Impact on Employment in Michigan of Eliminating Personal Consumption Expenditures on Tobacco, by Major Sector, 1992 Through 2005

| | (1) Gross Tobacco-Related | (2) Gross Replacement | (3) Net | (4) State and Local | Private Sector | | |
Year	Jobs Lost	Jobs	Employment†	Government	(5) Retail	(6) Wholesale	(7) Other§
1992	−19,127	24,735	5608	−2445	−617	−364	9034
1995	−17,492	21,314	3822	−2123	−970	−441	7356
2000	−15,005	17,330	2325	−1773	−1058	−475	5631
2005	−14,091	15,569	1478	−1567	−1020	−457	4522

Breakdown of Net Employment by Sector (No. of Jobs)‡

† Column 3 = column 1 + column 2.
‡ Sum of columns 4 through 7 = column 3.
§ Services, manufacturing, transportation, communication, public utilities, finance, construction, and mining.

more substantial gains in employment in all other industries (services, manufacturing, transportation, communication, public utilities, finance, construction, and mining). . . .

Impact on Tax Revenues

Assuming that government replaced half of lost cigarette excise tax revenues by increasing other taxes (our base-case assumption), we estimated that if tobacco product sales had suddenly ceased, government revenues would have fallen by $126 million in 1992, 1.3% of discretionary state revenues for the year (ie, excluding earmarked revenues). Much of other tax revenues associated with tobacco product sales, considerably smaller in amount than excise tax revenues, would have been replaced automatically by revenues from sales of alternative purchases (ie, the state's sales tax) and taxes on related personal and business income. By the year 2005, with no explicit program to replace more than half of cigarette taxes, the loss of government revenue would fall to $86 million (also in 1992 dollars). The reduced losses would be a result of the declining trend in tobacco purchases, along with a small contribution from the expanding economy associated with nontobacco expenditures.

Had the state chosen not to replace any lost excise tax, government revenues would have fallen by $254 million, or 2.6% of state government revenues. By 2005, the loss would have fallen to $167 million.

Doubling the Rate of Decline

Table 2 presents the results from the simulation of the more realistic scenario: a doubling of the expected rate of decline in tobacco product purchases, from 2.75% per person per year to 5.5%. The gross number of tobacco-related jobs that would be lost as a result of this greater than expected rate of decrease ranges from 1066 in 1992 to 4842 in the year 2005 (column 1). Gross replacement jobs, reflecting alternative spending of this money, are given in column 2. The net impact on employment in the state associated with the increased rate of decline in smok-

Table 2.—Gross and Net Impact on Employment in Michigan of Reducing Personal Consumption Expenditures on Tobacco, by Major Sector, 1992 Through 2005

| | (1) Gross Tobacco-Related | (2) Gross Replacement | (3) Net | (4) State and Local | Breakdown of Net Employment by Sector (No. of Jobs)‡ | | |
| | | | | | Private Sector | | |
Year	Jobs Lost	Jobs	Employment†	Government	(5) Retail	(6) Wholesale	(7) Other§
1992	−1066	1378	312	−137	−34	−20	503
1995	−2368	2919	551	−290	−122	−56	1019
2000	−3856	4622	766	−451	−226	−106	1549
2005	−4842	5633	791	−539	−301	−144	1775

† Column 3 = column 1 + column 2.
‡ Sum of columns 4 through 7 = column 3.
§ Services, manufacturing, transportation, communication, public utilities, finance, construction, and mining.

ing is seen in column 3: 312 more jobs in 1992, rising to 791 more jobs by 2005. The distribution of job losses and gains among industries, columns 4 through 7, reflects the same general pattern (albeit with much smaller numbers) as in the case of the complete elimination of tobacco product spending.

Replacement of half of lost cigarette excise tax revenues would have resulted in a net loss of $7 million in government revenues in Michigan in 1992 (less than 0.1% of discretionary state revenues), growing to $29.5 million in 2005. Had the state made no attempt to compensate for cigarette excise tax losses, government revenues would have fallen by $14 million in 1992 (0.14% of state revenues) and $59 million in 2005. . . .

Increasing Employment

We estimated both the gross and net economic implications of tobacco for the state of Michigan. Our estimate of the gross number of direct jobs, associated primarily with tobacco product wholesaling and retailing, is very close to the tobacco industry's most recent estimate: 7843 jobs in 1992 according to our analysis, 7724 in 1990 according to the Price Waterhouse analysis for the industry [*The Economic Impact of the Tobacco Industry on the United States Economy*]. The proximity of the two estimates suggests that both studies are measuring the same phenomenon. (Our estimates of indirect and induced employment, and hence total employment, are not comparable to those of Price Waterhouse, since the latter include the impact of tobacco spending nationwide on employment in Michigan, including, for example, the effects on Michigan employment of car buying by recipients of tobacco spending in the other 49 states.)

Unlike our analysis, none of the industry-sponsored studies evaluated the net economic impact of tobacco. However, one of the contractors [Chase Econometrics] acknowledged that money not spent on tobacco products would be reallocated to other spending, and that nationwide (combining tobacco and nontobacco states), the economic results with and without tobacco "would be substantially the same."

We found that, in a nontobacco state such as Michigan, expenditures on tobacco products actually decrease employment. The important corollary is that tobacco-control policies that succeed in reducing smoking in a nontobacco state may have a salutary effect on employment within the state, in addition to the obvious health benefits. . . .

> *"The industry's estimates greatly exaggerate tobacco's economic importance."*

Tobacco-Related Health Care

Neither the tobacco industry's analysis nor ours includes economic activity in the health care sector in estimating the economic contribution of tobacco. To be consistent with the industry's studies, we adopted their implicit assumption that the health effects of smoking are not relevant to the analysis. Clearly, this is an unreasonable assumption, producing a substantial underestimation of the gross impact of tobacco on employment. In Michigan, spending on tobacco-related health care was, conservatively, close to $2 billion in 1992, similar in magnitude to direct spending on tobacco products of approximately $1.8 billion. Thus, by producing illness, tobacco generated economic activity (jobs and incomes) in the health care industry in Michigan, just as it did in tobacco industry retailing and wholesaling. Indeed, tobacco-related health care may have accounted for more jobs in Michigan than did tobacco product sales per se, since half of the expenditures on the latter "leaked" out of state.

> *"Money not spent on tobacco products would be reallocated to other spending."*

Since the tobacco industry's economic argument asserts that a state will suffer economically if tobacco consumption declines, a complete examination of the issue would include consideration of the economic implications of the eventual elimination of tobacco-related disease. While we have not estimated this impact quantitatively, we can offer the following qualitative conclusions:

• Even if tobacco expenditures could cease instantaneously, tobacco-related health care expenditures would decline only gradually, since current tobacco-related disease reflects the cumulative effects of past decades of smoking.

• Just as in the case of tobacco product expenditures per se, reduced spending on tobacco-related health care would be redistributed to other spending within the economy that would generate "replacement" employment. Whether this alternative spending pattern would create more or fewer jobs depends on a number of interindustry factors. The alternative spending pattern likely would not create as many more jobs as would the direct reduction in spending on tobacco, however, since proportionately less health care spending in Michigan is exported to other states.

• The eventual absence of tobacco-related disease implies that, on average, Michigan residents would not contract serious illnesses until later in their (longer) lives. Therefore, some of the reduction in health care services realized in a tobacco-free state would translate into other kinds of health care services later on (possibly more geriatric medicine, for example), mitigating the diminution of the health care sector implied above. On balance, however, aggregate tobacco-related health care expenditures would be expected to fall, freeing resources to be reallocated to other uses.

Tobacco in Context

Ignoring the health care expenditures related to tobacco consumption, we estimate that tobacco product sales in Michigan were associated with approximately 19,000 jobs in the state in 1992, as well as more than $300 million in government revenues. Out of context, these are impressive-sounding numbers, especially to bureaucrats and legislators who must grapple with the difficult twin challenges of unemployment and perpetually strained government budgets. In context, however, the numbers are less impressive: they mask the fact that, on balance, expenditures on tobacco products actually reduce employment in the state. If consumers spent their money on goods and services other than tobacco products, the state would gain jobs.

The truly important consideration, however, is the one that places tobacco's economic role into a proper social context. Annually, tobacco claims the lives of more than 15,000 Michigan citizens. For the nation as a whole, the 1990 death toll was 419,000 Americans, each of whom lost an average of 12 years of life expectancy; millions of others suffer illness and disability as a direct consequence of smoking. Surely, any reasonable accounting of tobacco's "contribution" would emphasize the enormity of the health toll, with the economic consequences constituting no more than a distant secondary consideration.

> *"Expenditures on tobacco products actually decrease employment."*

When that secondary consideration is raised, however, it is essential that it be correctly interpreted: as this viewpoint has demonstrated, the industry's economic argument is misleading. In Michigan and, by extension, in other, perhaps all, of the more than 40 nontobacco states, tobacco-control policies can increase employment at the same time that they improve the public's health.

Smoking Should Not Be Regulated

by Jacob Sullum

About the author: *Jacob Sullum is the senior editor of* Reason, *a monthly libertarian magazine.*

In the introduction to the first major American book on public health, U.S. Army surgeon John S. Billings explained the field's concerns: "Whatever can cause, or help to cause, discomfort, pain, sickness, death, vice, or crime—and whatever has a tendency to avert, destroy, or diminish such causes—are matters of interest to the sanitarian; and the powers of science and the arts, great as they are, are taxed to the uttermost to afford even an approximate solution to the problems with which he is concerned."

Today's Issues

Despite this ambitious mandate—and the book's impressive length (nearly 1,500 pages in two volumes)—*A Treatise on Hygiene and Public Health* had little to say about the issues that occupy today's public health professionals. There were no sections on smoking, alcoholism, drug abuse, obesity, vehicular accidents, mental illness, suicide, homicide, domestic violence, or unwanted pregnancy. Published in 1879, the book was instead concerned with such things as compiling vital statistics, preventing the spread of disease, abating public nuisances, and assuring wholesome food, clean drinking water, and sanitary living conditions.

A century later, public health textbooks discuss the control of communicable diseases mainly as history. The field's present and future lie elsewhere. "The entire spectrum of 'social ailments,' such as drug abuse, venereal disease, mental illness, suicide, and accidents, includes problems appropriate to public health activity," explains Jack Smolensky in *Principles of Community Health* (1977). "The greatest potential for improving the health of the American people is to be found in what they do and don't do to and for themselves." Similarly, *Introduc-*

tion to Public Health (1978), by Daniel M. Wilner, Rosabelle Price Walkley, and Edward J. O'Neill, notes that the field, which once "had much narrower interests," now "includes the *social and behavioral aspects of life*—endangered by contemporary stresses, addictive diseases, and emotional instability."

A Striking Change

The extent of the shift can be sensed by perusing a few issues of the American Public Health Association's journal. In 1911, when the journal was first published, typical articles included "Modern Methods of Controlling the Spread of Asiatic Cholera," "Sanitation of Bakeries and Restaurant Kitchens," and "The Need of Exact Accounting for Still-Births." Issues published in 1995 offered "Menthol vs. Nonmenthol Cigarettes: Effects on Smoking Behavior," "Correlates of College Student Binge Drinking," and "Violence by Male Partners Against Women During the Childbearing Year: A Contextual Analysis." The journal also covers strictly medical issues, of course, and even runs articles on traditional public health topics such as vaccination, nutrition, and infant mortality. But the amount of space taken up by studies of social problems and behavioral issues is striking.

In a sense, the change in focus is understandable. After all, Americans are not dying the way they once did. The chapter on infant mortality in *A Treatise on Hygiene and Public Health* reports that during the late 1860s and early 1870s, two-fifths to one-half

> *"The public health establishment has become the most influential lobby for . . . control over Americans' personal choices."*

of children in major American cities died before reaching the age of 5. The major killers included measles, scarlet fever, smallpox, diphtheria, whooping cough, bronchitis, pneumonia, tuberculosis, and "diarrheal diseases." Largely because of such afflictions, life expectancy at birth was only 49 in 1900, compared to roughly 75 today, while the annual death rate was 17 per 1,000, compared to about half that today. Beginning in the 1870s, the discovery that infectious diseases were caused by specific microorganisms made it possible to control them through vaccination, antibiotics, better sanitation, water purification, and elimination of carriers such as rats and mosquitoes. At the same time, improvements in nutrition and living conditions increased resistance to infection. Although it is difficult to separate the effects of public health programs from the effects of rising affluence and changing patterns of work, there's no question that disease-control efforts have had an important impact on the length and quality of life.

Americans no longer live in terror of smallpox or cholera. Despite occasional outbreaks of infectious diseases such as rabies and tuberculosis, the fear of epidemics that was once an accepted part of life is virtually unknown. The one major exception is AIDS, which is not readily transmitted and remains largely confined to a few high-risk groups. For the most part, Americans die of things you can't catch: cancer, heart disease, trauma. Accordingly, the public health establishment is focusing on those causes and the factors underlying them. Having vanquished most true epidemics, it has turned its attention to metaphorical "epidemics" such as smoking, obesity, and suicide. Along the way, the public health establishment has become the most influential lobby for ever-increasing government control over Americans' personal choices. . . .

Official Nags

The concerns of public health practitioners have a way of influencing public policy. Surgeons general of the U.S. Public Health Service have become official nags, urging us to shape up so we can reach the health goals they have set for the nation. The wide domain of public health allows them to champion whatever causes interest them. C. Everett Koop said we should achieve "a smoke-free society" by the year 2000. Antonia Novello condemned liquor and beer advertising that she found distasteful. Joycelyn Elders pontificated about gun control and masturbation. The circumstances of Elders's departure and the battle over her successor show that both liberals and conservatives take the top public health job quite seriously.

The key event that elevated the surgeon general's prestige and visibility occurred in 1964, when Luther M. Terry released the report of his Advisory Committee on Smoking and Health. The document, which declared that "cigarette smoking is a health hazard of sufficient importance in the United States to warrant appropriate remedial action," heralded the decline of the U.S. tobacco industry and the beginning of the contemporary anti-smoking movement. It helped put risky behavior at the top of the public health agenda. . . .

Smoking as a Disease

In the public health literature, smoking is not an activity or even a habit. It is "the greatest community health hazard," "the single most important preventable cause of death," "the plague of our time," "the global tobacco epidemic." The disease metaphor has been used so much that it is now taken literally. The foreword to the 1988 surgeon general's report on nicotine addiction informs us,

> *"The concerns of public health practitioners have a way of influencing public policy."*

"Tobacco use is a disorder which can be remedied through medical attention." This definition was not always so casually accepted. In the 1977 monograph, *Tobacco Use as a Mental Disorder*, published by the National Institute on Drug Abuse, Jerome H. Jaffe noted that "a behavior that merely predisposes to other medical illnesses is not necessarily, in and of itself, a disease or disorder. . . . We certainly would not want to consider skiing as a mental disorder, although it clearly raises the likelihood of developing several

169

well-defined orthopedic disorders. Risk taking, *per se*, is not a mental disorder."

Yet today public health professionals consider smoking itself a disease, something inherently undesirable that happens to unwilling victims. "Free will is not within the power of most smokers," writes former CDC [Centers for Disease Control] Director William Foege in "The Growing Brown Plague," a 1990 editorial in the *Journal of the American Medical Association* (*JAMA*). If it were, they certainly would choose not to smoke. As Scott Ballin, chairman of the Coalition on Smoking OR Health, explains, "The product has no potential benefits. . . . It's addictive, so people don't have the choice to smoke or not to smoke."

These statements are part of a catechism intended to explain why so many people continue to smoke,

> *"Smoking might offer some people benefits that in their minds outweigh its hazards."*

when clearly they shouldn't. That catechism does not admit the possibility that smoking might offer some people benefits that in their minds outweigh its hazards. This blindness is inherent in the public health perspective, which seeks collective prescriptions that do not take account of individual tastes and preferences. It recognizes one supreme value—health—that cannot be trumped by other considerations.

Cigarette Advertising

Having promoted smoking from risk factor to disease, the public health establishment now targets alleged risk factors for smoking, most notably cigarette advertising. "If exposure to cigarette advertising is a risk factor for disease," writes Rep. Henry Waxman (D-Calif.) in a 1991 *JAMA* editorial, "it is incumbent on the public and elected officials to deal with it as we would the vector of any other pathogen." In other words, banning cigarette ads is like draining the swamps where the mosquitoes that carry malaria breed. That seems to be the assumption underlying . . . proposed restrictions on tobacco advertising.

The alarm about the danger posed by cigarette advertising is based largely on well-publicized studies in medical journals that prove less than the researchers' conclusions and accompanying editorials imply. A typical example is the 1991 *JAMA* study. The researchers reported that 6-year-olds were as likely to match Joe Camel with a pack of cigarettes as they were to match the Disney Channel logo with Mickey Mouse. "Given the serious consequences of smoking," they wrote, "the exposure of children to environmental tobacco advertising may represent an important health risk. . . ." But recognizing Joe Camel is not tantamount to smoking, any more than recognizing the logos for Ford and Chevrolet (which most of the kids in the study did) is tantamount to driving.

The same issue of *JAMA* carried an article reporting that Camel's market share among smokers under the age of 18 increased from 0.5 percent in 1988 to nearly 33 percent in 1991. The authors attributed the change to the Joe Camel campaign and concluded that "a total ban of tobacco advertising and promotions . . . can be based on sound scientific reasoning." Yet during the period covered by the study, smoking among minors actually *fell*. So while Joe Camel may have had something to do with the shift in brand preferences (a shift that also occurred in other age groups, though less dramatically), he cannot be blamed for convincing more kids to smoke.

Jean J. Boddewyn, a marketing professor at Baruch College who is skeptical of the alleged link between tobacco advertising and consumption levels, has argued that medical journals are not an appropriate venue for such research. Writing in the December 1993 issue of the *Journal of Advertising*, he suggests that medical editors and reviewers lack expertise in the area and are too quick to publish articles that reflect badly on the tobacco industry. "How would the [*Journal of Advertising*'s] reputation fare," he wonders, "if it published an article on the *health consequences of smoking*, after asking only advertising specialists to review it?" Boddewyn also complains that articles on tobacco advertising in medical journals rarely refer to relevant sources outside the public health literature. . . .

Treating Adults Like Children

The public health research on . . . "unhealthy" behavior is driven by the expectation that people will change their ways once they realize the risks they are taking. *Healthy People* [the 1979 surgeon general's report] notes that "formidable obstacles" stand in the way of improved public health. "Prominent among them are individual attitudes toward the changes necessary for better health," it says. "Though opinion polls note greater interest in healthier lifestyles, many people remain apathetic and unmotivated. . . . Some consider activities to promote health moralistic rather than scientific; still others are wary of measures which they feel may infringe on personal liberties. However, *the scientific basis for suggested measures has grown so compelling, it is likely that such biases will begin to shift*." (Emphasis added.) In other words, only those ignorant of the scientific evidence could possibly oppose the public health agenda.

"Joe Camel . . . cannot be blamed for convincing more kids to smoke."

This assumption is central to the public health mentality. Back in 1879, John S. Billings stated it quite candidly: "By some writers, as Wilhelm von Humboldt and John Stuart Mill, it is denied that the State should directly attempt to improve the physical welfare of its citizens, on the ground that such interference will probably do more harm than good. But all admit that the State should extend special protection to those who are incapable of judging their own best interests, or of taking care of themselves, such as the insane, persons of feeble intellect, or children; and we have seen that in sanitary matters the public at large are thus incompetent."

Billings was defending traditional public health measures aimed at preventing the spread of infectious diseases and controlling health hazards such as rotting animal carcasses. It is reasonable to expect that such measures will be welcomed by the intended beneficiaries, once they understand the aim. The same cannot be said of public health's new targets. Even when they know about the relevant hazards (and assuming the information is accurate), many people will continue to smoke, drink, take illegal drugs, eat fatty foods, buy guns, speed, eschew seat belts and motorcycle helmets, and otherwise behave in ways frowned upon by the public health establishment. This is not because they misunderstand; it's because, for the sake of pleasure, utility, or convenience, they are prepared to accept the risks. When public health experts assume that these decisions are wrong, they do indeed treat adults like incompetent children.

> *"The public health establishment seeks government power to impose its vision of virtue on the rest of America."*

One such expert, writing in the *New England Journal of Medicine* 20 years ago, declared, "It is a crime to commit suicide quickly. However, to kill oneself slowly by means of an unhealthy life style is readily condoned and even encouraged." The article prompted a response from Robert F. Meenan, a professor at the University of California School of Medicine in San Francisco, who observed: "Health professionals are trained to supply the individual with medical facts and opinions. However, they have no personal attributes, knowledge, or training that qualifies them to dictate the preferences of others. Nevertheless, doctors generally assume that the high priority that they place on health should be shared by others. They find it hard to accept that some people may opt for a brief, intense existence full of unhealthy practices. Such individuals are pejoratively labeled 'noncompliant' and pressures are applied on them to reorder their priorities."

Health or Virtue

More than 75 years ago, H.L. Mencken complained about this tendency to impose a moral value—the paramount importance of health—in the guise of medical science. "Hygiene is the corruption of medicine by morality," he wrote in 1919. "It is impossible to find a hygienist who does not debase his theory of the healthful with a theory of the virtuous." The public health establishment seeks government power to impose its vision of virtue on the rest of America.

And public health doctrine admits no limits. *Principles of Community Health* tells us that "the most widely accepted definition of individual health is that of the World Health Organization: 'Health is a state of complete physical, mental, and social well-being and not merely the absence of disease or infirmity.'" A government empowered to maximize "health" is a totalitarian government.

In response to such concerns, the public health establishment argues that government intervention is justified because individual decisions about risk affect other people. . . . This familiar line of reasoning implies that all resources—including not just taxpayer-funded welfare and health care but private savings, insurance coverage, and charity—are part of a common pool owned by "society as a whole" and guarded by the government. . . .

As Faith T. Fitzgerald, a professor at the University of California, Davis, Medical Center, writes in the *New England Journal of Medicine*: "Both health care providers and the commonweal now have a vested interest in certain forms of behavior, previously considered a person's private business, if the behavior impairs a person's 'health.' Certain failures of self-care have become, in a sense, crimes against society, because society has to pay for their consequences. . . . In effect, we have said that people owe it to society to stop misbehaving, and we use illness as evidence of misbehavior."

Most public health practitioners would presumably recoil at the full implications of the argument that government should override individual decisions affecting health because such decisions have an impact on "society as a whole." They are no doubt surprised and offended to be called "health fascists," when their goal is to extend and improve people's lives. But some defenders of the public health movement recognize that its aims are fundamentally collectivist and cannot be reconciled with the American tradition of limited government. In 1975 Dan E. Beauchamp, then an assistant professor of public health at the University of North Carolina and currently a professor in the School of Public Health at the State University of New York at Albany, presented a paper at the annual meeting of the American Public Health Association in which he argued that "the radical individualism inherent in the market model" is the biggest obstacle to improving public health.

> *"Of all the risk factors for disease and injury, freedom may be the most important."*

"The historic dream of public health that preventable death and disability ought to be minimized is a dream of social justice," Beauchamp said. "We are far from recognizing the principle that death and disability are collective problems and that all persons are entitled to health protection." He rejected "the ultimately arbitrary distinction between voluntary and involuntary hazards" and complained that "the primary duty to avert disease and injury still rests with the individual." He called upon public health practitioners to challenge "the powerful sway market-justice holds over our imagination, granting fundamental freedom to all individuals to be left alone." Of all the risk factors for disease and injury, freedom may be the most important.

A Tobacco Tax Increase Is Not Justified

by Jane Gravelle and Dennis Zimmerman

About the authors: *Jane Gravelle and Dennis Zimmerman are economists at the Congressional Research Service of the Library of Congress in Washington, D.C.*

American taxpayers seemed to disagree on almost everything about President Clinton's health care reform package, with one notable exception. A vast majority favored the proposed 75-cent tax on a pack of cigarettes. Were one to be cynical, such support might be explained by the fact that only about a quarter of adult Americans smoke, so that the majority of us anticipate receiving health care paid for by others. Fortunately, a more charitable—and conventional—explanation exists: that the 25 percent of American adults who smoke impose great costs on nonsmokers, thus a 75-cent tax increase would compensate nonsmokers for these social, or "external," costs. If true, nonsmokers can rest easy knowing that imposition of a cigarette tax is not only in their financial best interest, but is also abundantly fair.

Smokers Pay Their Way

But is it, in fact, fair? Let's take a look at the evidence. The financial costs smokers impose on nonsmokers have been extensively examined in a 1991 study funded by the Rand Corp. Updating the study's midrange estimate to 1995 price levels yields a net external cost of smoking of 33 cents per pack. Since current federal, state and local taxes are 50 cents per pack or more on average, the Rand-sponsored study suggests that smokers are already paying more than their way.

These modest spillover costs may seem inexplicable in light of the assertions of organizations that advocate taxes far larger than 75 cents per pack. But the Rand study makes some critical distinctions many of those organizations don't acknowledge. For instance, the Rand study identifies all of the costs and benefits that smokers impose on others—and excludes the costs smokers pay for

Jane Gravelle and Dennis Zimmerman, "Up in Smoke," *Washington Post National Weekly Edition*, June 13–19, 1994. Reprinted with permission.

themselves. Thus, the study includes as external costs only that portion of smokers' excess medical expenditures (49 cents per pack) and sick leave costs (1 cent per pack) not paid by smokers, the higher life and fire insurance premiums due to smoking (7 and 3 cents per pack, respectively) and the lost tax revenue smokers would have paid to retirement and health programs had they not died prematurely (12 cents per pack).

Additionally, the authors of the Rand study include the offsetting savings that smokers' premature death provides to nonsmokers—an obvious but often overlooked factor. After all, the alternative to death from a smoking-related illness is not immortality and perfect health—it is later death, and perhaps from a more costly illness (netted out in the 49 cents per pack above) or larger nursing home costs (a 6-cent offset per pack). Nonsmokers may not realize it, but they also benefit from the pension and Social Security payments that are not paid to smokers who die prematurely (33 cents per pack).

Considering the Cost of Smoking

Is this an all-too-typical example of economists' insensitivity to the human element of public policy? Let us hasten to emphasize that counting such savings does not mean that premature death is beneficial to society; that would be absurd. Premature death is costly to smokers, who are, of course, part of society, even when condemned to puff in doorways. But the savings do reduce the costs imposed on others and must be accounted for in an attempt to measure this net external cost and the size of the tax that would fairly compensate for it.

The Rand estimate is not, of course, without uncertainties. Different data and assumptions about various financial costs would increase the 33 cents per pack figure, but others, equally valid, would decrease it. The discussion of net external costs would not be complete, however, without specific discussion of one item—the magnitude of external costs from *passive* smoking—that is not included in this 33-cent estimate.

Concerns about the possible health effects of passive smoking have been heightened by the surgeon general's 1986 and the Environmental Protection Agency's 1992 reports linking lung cancer in adults and certain respiratory effects in children to second-hand smoke. Despite the positions taken by these government authorities, the extent of a passive smoking effect remains subject to dispute. The debate centers on whether exposure levels are large enough to cause an effect, statistical problems with the studies of effects in human populations, and new statistical studies with contradictory results.

"Smokers are already paying more than their way."

In any case, the lung cancer deaths pose a lifetime risk of only one-tenth to two-tenths of a percent and involve risks of the same order of magnitude as driving a small rather than a large car (the latter provides more protection in a crash than does the former). If a passive-smoking risk exists, it does not appear large enough to raise the 33-cent per pack estimated costs imposed by smokers on nonsmokers by more than a few cents per pack.

Even if we were to accept a much larger passive smoking effect, a tax might not be justified. If these effects occur within families, a higher tax would simply make family members financially worse off if their smoking member does not cease smoking in response to the tax (and available evidence suggests the vast majority of smokers will continue to smoke with a 75-cent tax).

The message is fairly clear. An increased tax based on the costs smokers impose on nonsmokers has not been justified. The evidence indicates that smokers are already paying, or possibly more than paying, their way.

Bad Choices

Nonsmokers might also justify the tax as being in the best interests of smokers. If smokers are making bad choices, if they are ignorant and irrational in adopting and continuing a habit that hurts them, should not a tax be used to discourage them?

Ignorance does not appear to be a significant problem. Although some respondents to surveys do not appear to accept the hazards of smoking, on average people actually overstate the mortality risks of smoking. These perceptions are documented in a book by Kip Viscusi, "Smoking: Making the Risky Decision." It is common for individuals to overstate the risks of highly publicized dangers. Although smokers perceive on average somewhat smaller risks than nonsmokers (a 47 percent lifetime risk of eventually dying from a smoking-related illness rather than a 59 percent risk), those perceptions are considerably larger than the real risks suggested by scientific evidence (an 18 to 36 percent risk). Notably, teenagers actually perceive higher risks than do older individuals, perhaps because their exposure to health information is more recent.

Could smokers, even though they are intellectually aware of the dangers, be making irrational decisions? This appears to be the only altruistic argument remaining for nonsmokers to justify increasing the cigarette tax. Economists have long noted that individuals engage in many activities that are risky or hazardous to health—working at risky jobs, engaging in risky sports, following less than ideal diets—but which are not normally characterized as irrational. Thus, indulgence in an unhealthy or risky activity is not necessarily evidence of a need for the government to intervene; were it so, intervention in a whole range of activities would be justified.

"An increased tax based on the costs smokers impose on nonsmokers has not been justified."

The argument specific to cigarettes is that nicotine is addictive; therefore smokers are unable to change their behavior. Moreover, individuals typically begin experimenting with smoking when they are young, and thus may not be aware of the difficulty of quitting in the future. This issue is difficult to grapple with, especially since the term "addiction" is such an emotionally charged one, conjuring up the vision of physical enslavement.

Considering Addiction

What do we know about the behavior of smokers in the face of the habit-forming nature of tobacco consumption? From one perspective, the majority of smokers say they would like to quit or wish they had not started. Most start when they are young, many fail when they try to quit, and a large fraction of teenagers who smoke say they expect to quit in a few years, yet do not.

From another perspective, many smokers have been successful in quitting (there are as many former smokers as there are current smokers). Evidence on the responsiveness of smokers to changes in price indicates a response typical of many other commodities, and publicity about health effects did reduce smoking substantially. Survey evidence suggests that people, including teenagers, are aware that it is difficult to quit smoking. Moreover, the pattern of wishing to change and failing to do so applies equally well—or perhaps even better—to a wide range of other behaviors such as losing weight or getting in shape with an exercise program. Although the reasons for failure may be different than is the case for smoking, here too individuals wish to change, yet abandon attempts to do so.

> *"The evidence . . . does not provide nonsmokers a convincing economic rationale for support of an increase in the cigarette tax."*

Unlike the external cost and risk assessment issues already discussed, this addiction issue is hard to resolve. Perhaps practicalities should be determining. If there is a serious addiction problem preventing individuals from quitting, a tax may not be the best remedy because the most addicted individuals will presumably be the least responsive to a price increase.

The group of greatest concern is teenagers. Although evidence suggests a price increase will discourage teenage smoking initiation, the tax would penalize a much larger number of adult smokers (only 6 percent of smokers are adolescents). Perhaps approaches more targeted to the teenage population should be considered, such as better enforcement of laws prohibiting sales to minors and more educational programs about the addiction issue.

Of course, the decision to adopt a cigarette tax will reflect many perspectives, including revenue needs and political feasibility. And society does sometimes impose the preferences of the majority on the minority for reasons other than those stressed by economics. The evidence presented thus far, however, does not provide nonsmokers a convincing economic rationale for support of an increase in the cigarette tax.

Increasing Tobacco Taxes Would Harm the Poor

by John Stamm

About the author: *John Stamm is a public policy analyst for the Tax Equity Alliance for Massachusetts in Boston.*

Since Surgeon General Luther Terry released the first official warnings in 1964, smoking in the United States has been steadily declining. But surveys have consistently shown this decline to be smaller and slower among less-educated Americans.

Studies done for the Centers for Disease Control detail these trends. While smoking decreased across all groups between 1974 and 1984, the percentage of college graduates who smoked declined almost five times faster than that of the rest of society. By 1985 18% of college graduates smoked, versus 34% of those who didn't graduate from high school. Most (60%) college graduates who had ever smoked had quit. Only 40% of high school graduates or dropouts had kicked the habit.

Using this data to project American smoking trends to the year 2000, researchers found the education gap widening. They predicted that more than 30% of Americans who do not continue their education past high school will be smoking in the 21st century, while less than 10% of college graduates will still be lighting up. This three-to-one ratio led the authors to conclude that "smoking in the U.S. is increasingly becoming a behavior primarily of the less educated and the socioeconomically disadvantaged."

Because more people who have less money to pay for the habit are smoking, you would be hard pressed to design a tax that hits our poorest families harder [than does a cigarette tax]. Numbers published by the Congressional Budget Office show that, on average, families in the lowest-earning fifth spend, as a percentage of income, nearly 8 times more on cigarettes than the wealthiest fifth. . . .

The poor have already endured years of state excise hikes. Unable to run

Excerpted from John Stamm, "Butting Heads over the Tobacco Tax," *Dollars & Sense*, June 1993. Reprinted with permission from *Dollars & Sense*, a progressive economics magazine published six times a year. First-year subscriptions cost $18.95 and may be ordered by writing to *Dollars & Sense*, One Summer St., Somerville, MA 02143.

deficits and faced with voter hostility toward income and property taxes, state and local governments in budget crises have increasingly relied on sales taxes, sin taxes, and fees. Between 1985 and 1990, there were 22 separate increases in state sales taxes and 62 separate increases in state cigarette excises. These increases have piled further demands on the poor just as their real incomes have fallen. On average nationwide, lower- and middle-income families pay three to four times more of their income on sales and excise taxes than the wealthy, while the poorest 20% spend seven times as much on such taxes as the richest 25%. . . .

The Sinners Shall Pay

Both Bill and Hillary Clinton have cited the costs smokers impose on the rest of society as a reason for a high cigarette tax. . . . When asked about "sin" taxes and their effects on lower- and middle-class Americans, Clinton said, "I think that we are spending a ton of money in private insurance and in government taxpaying to deal with the health care problems occasioned by bad health habits, and particularly smoking."

This concern for what smokers do to the rest of society, not just to themselves, has emerged recently as federal decision-makers' favorite reason to tax smokers. But estimates of these costs—particularly those cited by Clinton and other politicians—fail to separate costs smokers impose on others from the damage they cause themselves. Many studies, such as the oft-cited Office of Technology Assessment 1985 analysis, which estimated annual costs as high as $65 billion, add together both social and personal costs.

But another extensive study, done by Willard G. Manning and a group of economists for the University of Michigan in 1989, focused only on the costs to the rest of "us"—the expenses Clinton means by "a ton of money." Adding up the costs of medical bills, fire damage, and lost output due to sickness, the Rand study found that smokers already pay these costs in the current state and federal excises. Key to this finding is the rather grim truth that, by dying young and quickly, smokers give society their most productive years and leave behind unreceived pension and social security payments.

> *"Smoking in the U.S. is increasingly becoming a behavior primarily of the less educated."*

The distinction between social and personal costs is key to judging Clinton's stand on sin taxes. To sell the tax to the general public, he has emphasized the need to get sinners back for what they're doing to the rest of us. If that's justice, it's already done.

Policy, Not Punishment

Some have argued that funnelling revenues back into low-income communities would offset the regressivity of the tobacco tax. Legislative maneuvering could easily derail efforts to do that, but even if they were successful the tax would still follow the tax path of least resistance and dig deeper into the pockets of our least-educated and least-compensated citizens. There is no erasing its initial regressive impact.

Better arguments in favor of the tax focus on consumption: the potential for curbing smoking is any tobacco tax's greatest asset. But it's possible to value its power to save lives and still ask how many, who will pay the price, and whether we have alternatives.

First of all, it's difficult to predict precise effects on consumption. Smaller excise hikes have reduced the number of smokers by a wide range of 4–7% for every 10% rise in price. If Clinton were to double the price of cigarettes, we could see anywhere from 4 to 7 out of every 10 smokers quit or not start as a result—and anywhere from 3 to 6 smokers left paying the hefty tab.

These projected reductions are small compared to the enormous success public officials and antismoking activists have already realized with methods that do not punish: thirty years of government warnings, advertising restrictions, anti-smoking advertising and education, and restrictions on smoking in public spaces. A 1989 report published in the *American Journal of Public Health* concluded that "in the absence of the anti-smoking campaign, adult per capita cigarette consumption in 1987 would have been an estimated 79–89% higher." The continued damage smoking causes shouldn't obscure the success of these efforts. With this campaign, we have been better able to reduce the damage caused by nicotine than that of any other drug—or any other self-destructive habit—in our society.

> *"You would be hard pressed to design a tax that hits our poorest families harder."*

Education—not coercion—is the best solution to our smoking ills. We must continue, and intensify, the thirty years of education we have begun. Progressives should not allow punishment to prevail.

Government Regulation of Smoking Threatens Constitutional Rights

by Malcolm Wallop

About the author: *Malcolm Wallop, a former Republican senator from Wyoming, is chairman of Frontiers for Peace, a public policy organization in Arlington, Virginia, that advocates private property rights and personal freedoms.*

Remember Aug. 10, 1995. On that day, a President of the United States used the U.S. Constitution for cheap political gain. On that day, the most sacred of all the amendments to the Constitution, the First Amendment, was forsworn by President Bill Clinton.

White House political gurus stuck their fingers in the air and concluded that there were more nonsmokers in America than smokers. Their simple-minded strategy: Let's get all the nonsmokers to vote for us. Big-government regulators, such as power-happy Food and Drug Administration Commissioner David Kessler, determined that the First Amendment was not a fundamental right but a simple notion obstructing their grand plan to wipe out an entire industry.

Cracking Down on Freedoms

It is not surprising that Clinton picked Kessler to be the point person in cracking down on constitutional freedoms. He's a pro at it.

More than 150,000 American heart attack patients have died because the FDA needlessly refused to approve a life-saving drug already approved in Europe. On average, in Europe, drugs are approved for use nearly six years earlier than in the United States. American consumers can't use life-saving drugs that are commonly used elsewhere because Kessler says *no*.

More than 50% of American medical device companies are moving jobs and manufacturing operations overseas because the FDA bureaucracy makes it so

Malcolm Wallop, "The Constitution and the Marlboro Man," *Los Angeles Times*, August 30, 1995. Reprinted with permission.

hard for them to make their products here.

And then there's the surgeon from Virginia who plans to travel to England for an operation to implant a shoulder device—a device that he invented but can't market here.

Kessler is a man with a mission, and it isn't our safety. Increase the size and scope of the FDA, establish an FDA police force, create a regulatory nightmare for any company looking to make a profit and withhold drugs from people who desperately need them to save their very lives—then you have real power.

Look out, Mr. President: Commissioner Kessler is choosing who lives and who dies. With your blessing, he is playing God.

Clinton is wrong. It is not a question of angry smokers and satisfied non-smokers. Both groups are Americans with rights. The American people will see this tobacco assault for what it really is: The government, once again, telling us what to do and what is best for us.

Well, sorry, folks, but the government has no idea what is good for you or for me. Furthermore, our government has no authority to infringe upon what I think is best for my life. There is consensus that smoking is a health hazard, but so too are hunting, parachuting, eating red meat, swimming alone, drinking alcohol and climbing mountains.

We Americans cherish our constitutional rights. We do not pick presidents to have them reduce those freedoms. Under the Constitution, the federal government has no standing whatsoever to make such decisions. How dare the government exercise power over us—power never granted to it in the first place.

This issue has nothing to do with tobacco. Tobacco happens to be the vehicle for more government intrusion into our lives.

For argument's sake, however, let's take a close look at how the President is setting aside the First Amendment to destroy an industry. He and Kessler are calling for a prohibition on using trade names of non-tobacco companies, such as Cartier, Ritz and Harley Davidson, to advertise a cigarette product as well as for a mandate that a corporate-sponsored event be named for the corporation and not a product. They also would dictate the parameters of advertisements.

If ever there was a definitive example of big versus limited government, it's Clinton's attack on the tobacco industry. Next, it could be beef or automobiles that inconvenience Clinton's rule.

Whether you like smoking or find it thoroughly disgusting, step back and look at the totality of what is being done without authority. Must Americans give up their rights simply because a liberal President and a big-government bureaucrat say that we must? Surely not.

The First Amendment to the Constitution is first because it protects us from tyrants. Our job now as citizens, smokers or nonsmokers, is to work within the political, public and legislative arenas to vote out of office those who believe our Constitution counts for nothing.

Bibliography

Books

American Heart Association	*Active and Passive Tobacco Exposure: A Serious Pediatric Health Problem*. Dallas: American Heart Association, 1994.
American Heart Association	*Public Policy on Smoking and Health: Toward a Smoke-Free Generation by the Year 2000*. Dallas: American Heart Association, 1986.
Canadian Council on Smoking and Health	*Taking Control: An Action Handbook on Women and Tobacco*. 2nd ed. Ottawa: Canadian Council on Smoking and Health, 1993.
Karen Casey	*If Only I Could Quit: Recovering from Nicotine Addiction*. Center City, MN: Hazelden, 1995.
Judith A. Douville	*Active and Passive Smoking Hazards in the Workplace*. New York: Van Nostrand Reinhold, 1990.
Jeanne E.	*Twelve Steps for Tobacco Users: For Recovering People Addicted to Nicotine*. Center City, MN: Hazelden, 1995.
Stanton A. Glantz et al.	*The Cigarette Papers*. Berkeley and Los Angeles: University of California Press, 1996.
Health Canada	*Tobacco Control: A Blueprint to Protect the Health of Canadians*. Ottawa: Ministry of National Health and Welfare, 1995.
Philip J. Hilts	*Smokescreen: The Truth Behind the Tobacco Industry Cover-Up*. Reading, MA: Addison-Wesley, 1996.
Institute of Medicine	*Growing Up Tobacco Free*. Washington, DC: National Academy Press, 1994.
Richard Kluger	*Ashes to Ashes: America's Hundred-Year Cigarette War, the Public Health, and the Unabashed Triumph of Philip Morris*. New York: Knopf, 1996.
Cheryl L. Lockett	*Smoking in the Workplace: A Review of Arbitrary Decisions*. Fort Washington, PA: LRP Publications, 1988.
Tom O'Connell	*Up in Smoke: The Nicotine Challenge in Recovery*. Center City, MN: Hazelden, 1995.
	and Health, 1988.
C. Tracy Orleans and John Slade, eds.	*Nicotine Addiction: Principles and Management*. New York: Oxford University Press, 1993.
Terry A. Rustin	*Quit and Stay Quit: A Personal Program to Stop Smoking*. Center City, MN: Hazelden, 1995.

Bibliography

Tobacco Institute	*An Assessment of the Current Legal Climate Concerning Smoking in the Workplace.* Washington, DC: Tobacco Institute, 1988.
Tobacco Institute	*Indoor Pollution: Is Your Workplace Making You Sick?* Washington, DC: Tobacco Institute, 1988.
Robert D. Tollison	*Clearing the Air: Perspective on Environmental Tobacco Smoke.* Lexington, MA: Lexington Books, 1988.

Periodicals

Carl E. Bartecchi, Thomas D. MacKenzie, Robert W. Schrier	"The Human Costs of Tobacco Use," Part I, *New England Journal of Medicine*, March 31, 1994.
Peter L. Berger	"Furtive Smokers—and What They Tell Us About America," *Commentary*, June 1994.
Dennis L. Breo	"Kicking Butts—AMA, Joe Camel, and the 'Black Flag' War on Tobacco," *JAMA*, October 27, 1993.
Congressional Digest	"Second-Hand Tobacco Smoke," entire issue of congressional testimony, May 1994. Available from 3231 P St. NW, Washington, DC 20007.
Lowell C. Dale	"High-Dose Nicotine Patch Therapy," *JAMA*, November 1, 1995.
Clifford E. Douglas	"The Tobacco Industry's Use of Nicotine as a Drug," *Priorities*, vol. 6, no. 2, 1994. Available from the American Council on Science and Health, 1995 Broadway, 2nd Fl., New York, NY 10023-5860.
Jonathan Franzen	"Sifting the Ashes," *New Yorker*, May 13, 1996.
Alix M. Freedman	"Cigarette Defector Says CEO Lied to Congress About View of Nicotine," *Wall Street Journal*, January 26, 1996.
Elizabeth Gleick	"Tobacco Blues," *Time*, March 11, 1996.
JAMA	Entire section on tobacco use, April 24, 1996.
Holman W. Jenkins Jr.	"Tobacco Wars: A Study in Disingenuousness," *Wall Street Journal*, January 2, 1996.
Kai Maristen	"Nicotine, an Autobiography," *American Scholar*, Summer 1996.
Morton Mintz	"Blowing Smoke Rings Around the Statehouses," *Washington Monthly*, May 1996.
Mother Jones	Special report on the politics of tobacco, May/June 1996.
Steven Roberts	"Teens on Tobacco: Kids Smoke for Reasons All Their Own," *U.S. News & World Report*, April 18, 1994.
Brad Rodu and Philip Cole	"Would a Switch from Cigarettes to Smokeless Tobacco Benefit Public Health?" *Priorities*, vol. 7, no. 4, 1995.
Jane Buckley Smith	"Smoke Again and Live Again," *National Review*, December 11, 1995.
Wall Street Journal	"Cigarette Regulation Is Formally Proposed: Industry Sues to Halt It," August 11, 1995.
Kenneth E. Warner et al.	"Employment Implications of Declining Tobacco Product Sales for the Regional Economies of the United States," *JAMA*, April 24, 1996.

Organizations to Contact

The editors have compiled the following list of organizations concerned with the issues debated in this book. The descriptions are derived from materials provided by the organizations. All have publications or information available for interested readers. The list was compiled on the date of publication of the present volume; names, addresses, and phone and fax numbers may change. Be aware that many organizations take several weeks or longer to respond to inquiries, so allow as much time as possible.

Action on Smoking and Health
2013 H St. NW
Washington, DC 20006
(202) 659-4310
fax: (202) 833-3921

Action on Smoking and Health promotes the rights of nonsmokers against the harms of smoking. It provides scientific, educational, legal, and advocacy services, and it worked to ban tobacco ads from radio and television and to establish no-smoking sections on airplanes, trains, and buses. Action on Smoking and Health publishes the bimonthly newsletter *ASH Smoking and Health Review* and handouts on a variety of topics such as nicotine addiction, passive smoking, and the costs of workplace smoking.

American Cancer Society
316 Pennsylvania Ave. SE
Washington, DC 20003
(202) 546-4011
fax: (202) 546-1682

The American Cancer Society is one of the primary organizations in the United States devoted to educating the public about cancer and to funding cancer research. Because smoking can cause cancer, the society spends a great deal of its resources on educating the public about the harms of smoking and on lobbying for antismoking legislation. The American Cancer Society publishes hundreds of publications, from reports and surveys to position papers.

Americans for Nonsmokers' Rights
2530 San Pablo Ave., Suite J
Berkeley, CA 94702
(510) 841-3032
fax: (510) 841-7702

Americans for Nonsmokers' Rights seeks to protect the rights of nonsmokers in the workplace and other public settings. It maintains the American Nonsmokers' Rights Foundation, which promotes smoking prevention, nonsmokers' rights, and public education about passive smoking. The organization publishes the quarterly newsletter *ANR Update*, *Legislative Approaches to a Smokefree Society*, and *Matrix of Major Local Smoking Ordinances in the U.S.*

185

Citizens for a Tobacco-Free Society (CATS)
8660 Lynnehaven Dr.
Cincinnati, OH 45236
(513) 677-6666

CATS is made up of health and environmental organizations and individuals concerned with indoor air pollution caused by tobacco smoke. It seeks to create a tobacco-free society by the year 2000 and to this end supports a total ban on smoking in enclosed public places, restaurants, and workplaces. CATS serves as a resource center for the news media on smoking and health issues. It distributes information on the effects of second-hand smoke and how to lobby for laws to maintain clean indoor air. CATS publishes a quarterly newsletter and news report and a periodic news release.

Coalition on Smoking OR Health
1150 Connecticut Ave. NW, Suite 820
Washington, DC 20036
(202) 452-1184
fax: (202) 452-1417

Formed by the American Lung Association and the American Cancer Society, the coalition lobbies legislators to pass laws aimed at decreasing and preventing the use of tobacco. It supports increased cigarette taxes, stronger warnings on cigarette packages and advertisements, the banning of smoking in public buildings, and FDA regulation of the tobacco industry, among other measures. The coalition publishes the annual *Framework for Public Policy*, the quarterly newsletter *News from the Coalition*, the annual *State Legislated Actions on Tobacco Issues*, and other reports and pamphlets.

Group Against Smokers' Pollution (GASP)
PO Box 632
College Park, MD 20741-0632
(301) 459-4791

GASP is made up of nonsmokers adversely affected by tobacco smoke, who work to promote the rights of nonsmokers, to educate the public about the problems of second-hand smoke, and to encourage the regulation of smoking in public places. The organization provides information and referral services and distributes educational materials, buttons, posters, and bumper stickers. GASP publishes booklets and pamphlets such as *The Nonsmokers' Bill of Rights* and *The Nonsmokers' Liberation Guide*.

Smoker's Rights Alliance
20 E. Main St., Suite 710
Mesa, AZ 85201
(602) 461-8882

The alliance comprises individuals interested in preserving the right to smoke without interference from the government. It educates and informs members of their rights and lobbies to protect those rights. The alliance publishes the quarterly newsletter *Smoke Signals*.

Stop Teen-Age Addiction to Tobacco (STAT)
511 E. Columbus Ave.
Springfield, MA 01105
(413) 732-STAT
fax: (413) 732-4219

STAT works to raise public awareness of the role of tobacco advertisements and promotions in influencing children to smoke. It cooperates with merchants to prevent children from buying cigarettes. STAT conducts research, maintains a library and speakers bureau, and compiles statistics. It publishes the semiannual *Tobacco Free Youth Reporter* and the book *Sixty Years of Deception: An Analysis and Compilation of Cigarette Advertising from 1925–1985.*

Tobacco Merchants Association of the United States
PO Box 8019
Princeton, NJ 08543-8019
(609) 275-4900
fax: (609) 275-8379

The association represents manufacturers of tobacco products; tobacco leaf dealers, suppliers, and distributors; and others related to the tobacco industry. It tracks statistics on the sale and distribution of tobacco and informs its members of this information through the following periodicals: the weekly newsletters *Executive Summary*, *World Alert*, and *Tobacco Weekly*; the biweeklies *Leaf Bulletin* and *Legislative Bulletin*; the monthlies *Trademark Report*, *Tobacco Barometer: Smoking, Chewing & Snuff*, and *Tobacco Trade Barometer*; and the quarterly newsletter *Issues Monitor*. The association has a reference library and also offers online services and economic, statistical, media-tracking, legislative, and regulatory information.

Tobacco Products Liability Project
Northeastern University School of Law
400 Huntington Ave.
Boston, MA 02115
(617) 373-2026
fax: (617) 373-3672

The project's members include doctors, lawyers, public health officials, and academics who encourage product liability lawsuits against the marketers of tobacco products. The organization advocates for victims of tobacco-related diseases and injuries such as cancer and burns. It also discourages teenage smoking and publicizes the harmful effects of smoking on health. The project acts as an information clearinghouse and publishes the newsletter *Tobacco on Trial* in addition to reports and pamphlets.

Index